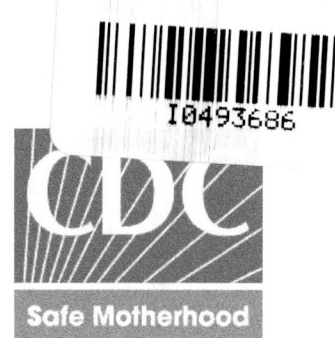

Safe Motherhood

I0493686

Questionnaire Design

Reproductive Health
Epidemiology Series
Module 4

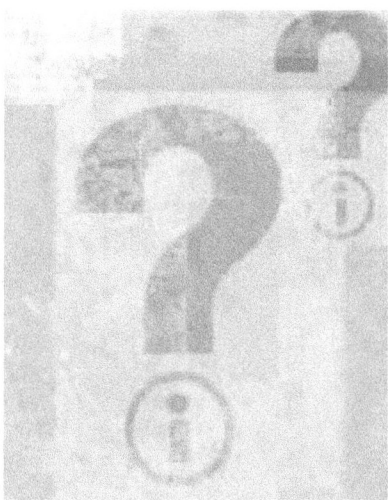

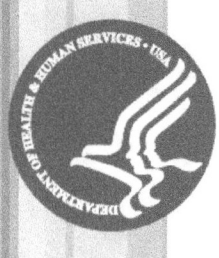

2003

U.S. DEPARTMENT OF HEALTH AND HUMAN SERVICES

QUESTIONNAIRE DESIGN

Reproductive Health
Epidemiology Series
Module 4

September 2003

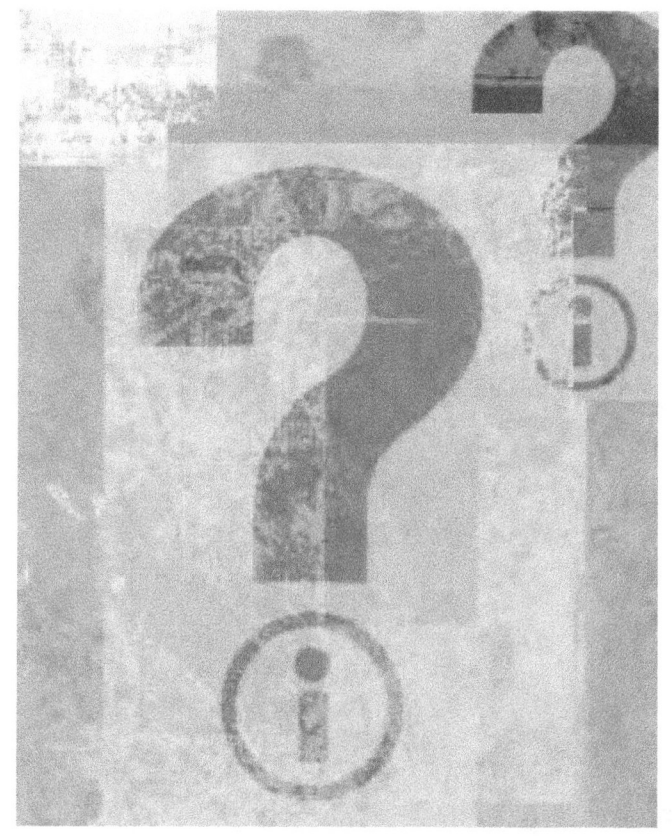

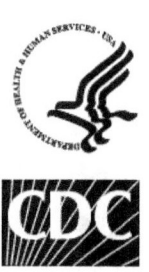

CDC

The United States Agency for International Development (USAID) provided funding for this project through a Participating Agency Service Agreement with CDC (936-3038.01).

Questionnaire Design

Jill A. McDonald, PhD
Nancy Burnett, BS
Victor G. Coronado, MD, MPH
Renee L. Johnson, MSPH

DEPARTMENT OF HEALTH AND HUMAN SERVICES
Centers for Disease Control and Prevention
National Center for Chronic Disease Prevention and Health Promotion
Division of Reproductive Health
Atlanta, Georgia, U.S.A.
2003

Contents

QUESTIONNAIRE DESIGN

LEARNING OBJECTIVES

This module is designed for reproductive health professionals who are interested in evaluating or designing questionnaires for use in epidemiologic studies and surveillance.

After studying the material in this module the student should be able to:

- Understand the importance of identifying the specific research question(s) under study before developing the questionnaire.

- Assess the adequacy and appropriateness of a questionnaire to answer particular research question(s).

- Discuss the factors to be considered in designing a questionnaire-based project, such as population size and budget.

- Determine possible modes of administration for the questionnaire.

- Describe the common pitfalls of questionnaire wording and construction that affect data quality.

- List the questions, codes, and units of measurement that will be used to create the specific variables needed to answer a research question.

- Develop the format and layout of a questionnaire.

- Develop a strategy to pretest a questionnaire and administration procedures.

- Describe the measures that should be taken to protect the confidentiality of the subjects responding to the questionnaire.

- Understand the implications of designing questionnaires for multicultural populations.

- Understand how and to what extent the validity and reliability of a questionnaire can be assessed.

SCOPE AND GOALS OF THIS CHAPTER

Questionnaire design is a cornerstone of epidemiologic methods, and the questionnaire is one of epidemiology's most valuable tools. The term *questionnaire* is variously defined by investigators *(1–3)*, but here refers to a structured document that is used to collect information from respondents about themselves or others. Once collected, the information is converted into measures of factors that are important to the research question under investigation. Although other data collection instruments, such as medical record abstraction forms, are not specifically covered in this chapter, many of the principles of questionnaire design pertain to them as well.

Questionnaires are essential in the collection of epidemiologic data that are difficult to obtain or not available elsewhere. In many investigations, the respondent may be the only source of information about his or her personal exposures, health-related behaviors, confounding factors, and other important variables of interest. In the Case-Control Study of Adolescent Pregnancy (Example 2.1 in Chapter 2: Developing a Research Proposal), for instance, respondent knowledge of fertility control practices, a factor that may be predictive of teen pregnancy, can be ascertained only from the couples participating in the study. Moreover, this kind of information can often be collected only indirectly through a series of questions because there is no single question that describes knowledge of fertility control practices.

In this chapter we will be focusing on the use of questionnaires to collect factual data, or data that are factual at least in theory. In the above example from Chapter 2, for example, the respondent either does or does not have knowledge of oral contraceptives; similarly, a respondent does or does not consume alcohol and has or has not been pregnant, etc. Outside of epidemiology, questionnaires are commonly used to collect other kinds of nonfactual data, such as information about attitudes and other sentiments that may be associated with health-related behavior *(4)*. Designing questions to collect these nonfactual data is a more difficult process and does not fall within the scope of this chapter. For guidance on the construction and testing of questions that measure sentiments and other psychological variables, readers should refer to the psychometric literature *(4,5)*.

Epidemiologic information collected through a questionnaire can be relatively objective and straightforward, such as the taking of a body measurement, or more subjective and complicated, such as the recalling and reporting of a past exposure. Regardless of the level of complexity, however, all questionnaire data are further complicated by measurement error. The measurement of body weight, for example, may be affected by use of differently calibrated scales and other differences in the weighing procedure, and the report of a past exposure may be affected by differences in the way the question is asked or interpreted. As shown in Figure 1, any given measurement obtained from questionnaire data almost certainly contains an element of error *(6)*.

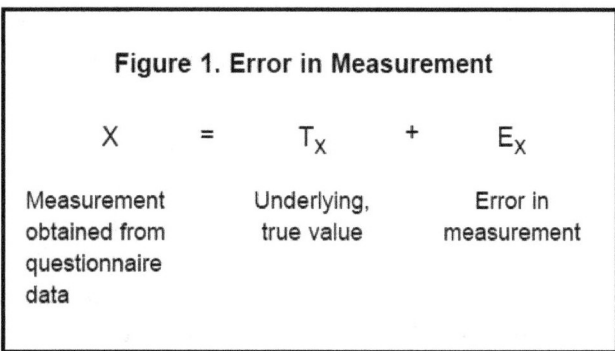

Figure 1. Error in Measurement

$$X \quad = \quad T_X \quad + \quad E_X$$

| Measurement obtained from questionnaire data | Underlying, true value | Error in measurement |

Measurement error, which can be random or systematic, leads to the misclassification of respondents regarding the risk factors, exposure, the disease under study, or all of these. A well-designed questionnaire aims to construct and standardize the questions that are asked of each respondent in such a way as to minimize error and the bias it may bring about. When measurement error is kept to a minimum, the inferences that can be drawn from questionnaire data about the true values in the study population are more valid and increase the likelihood that study results can be generalized to other populations *(7)*. Measurement error is not the only important source of bias in surveys, but it should be of highest concern to investigators. Unlike confounding and some forms of selection bias that can be corrected in analysis *(8)*, misclassification due to measurement error, especially when misclassification affects multiple variables, is impractical, if not impossible, to fix (Chapter 4: Epidemiologic Study Design).

Raw questionnaire data are the basic building blocks of study results, and the overall quality of study results can only be as high as the quality of the raw data on which they are based *(9)*.

In this chapter, we will focus on the ways in which the careful design and implementation of a questionnaire-based study can help prevent the occurrence of measurement error. Measurement error can arise from a number of interdependent sources, including problems in the design of the questions themselves, errors made by respondents, errors made by interviewers, and errors made in the abstracting, coding, and processing of the data. Figure 2 shows the common sources of measurement error.

Figure 2. Sources of Measurement Error

- Questionnaire design problems

- Respondent error

- Interviewer error

- Abstracting, coding, and processing error

Although we will touch on each of these sources, it is beyond the scope of this chapter to give them each the kind of attention they deserve. A well-designed questionnaire, however, will not only reduce measurement error in its own right, but will also serve as a critical first step in the prevention of error due to other sources as well.

Asking questions of respondents via questionnaire is a variation on the asking and answering of questions in everyday conversation, where certain expectations of speakers operate and govern the exchange of information *(10–12)* (Figure 3).

Figure 3. Expectations of Speakers in Everyday Conversation

- Speaker will choose language that is clearly understood by the listener.

- Speaker will provide only relevant information.

- Speaker will tell the truth.

- Speaker will not be redundant.

Investigators who are aware of these expectations and the ways they may influence the answers of respondents are better equipped to design questionnaires. In epidemiology, our goal is to turn the process of everyday conversation into one of rigorous measurement, and the questionnaire is our protocol for that conversation. We aim for a completely standardized exchange of information, where dialogue is unambiguous and task-oriented, and attention to quality control is ever present. At the same time, the process of completing a questionnaire should be a safe, interesting, and not unduly burdensome experience for the respondent.

A questionnaire should meet at least five general objectives to yield high-quality response data *(13)*.

1) Each question should be interpreted by different respondents in the same way and in a way that is consistent with what the investigator expected.

2) Each question should specify the type of answer expected.

3) Each question should ask something all respondents are able to provide.

4) Each question should ask something all respondents are willing to provide.

5) Each question should be administered to respondents in the same way.

Of course, even the most carefully crafted and administered questions that are successful in holding measurement error to a minimum will not assure data quality and validity of study results if, on the one hand, they are not the right questions to begin with *(14)*, and if, on the other, they are not processed and analyzed appropriately.

USE OF QUESTIONNAIRES IN RESEARCH

A questionnaire-based research study that collects personal information which can be linked to individual human subjects *(15)* must be designed and conducted in an ethical manner that protects the research subjects. (See *The Declaration of Helsinki*, page 6.) Various cultural considerations and standards may be applicable, depending on where the study is taking place. For example, study participants generally can be paid a reasonable reimbursement for their time and incidental expenses (e.g., transportation), but "the ethical propriety of such inducements...must be assessed in the light of the traditions of the culture" *(17)*. A payment that is appropriate in one setting may be unacceptably low, high, coercive, or otherwise inappropriate in another. The 1979 Belmont Report set ethical guidelines for protecting human research subjects in federally funded research *(18)*. Research funded completely or in part by the U.S. government must comply with the sections of the U.S. Code of Federal Regulations *(15)* that are based on the Belmont report.

Careful development and implementation of the research protocol and questionnaire are an underlying part of human subjects protection. Individuals should not be asked to participate in a study or survey that is seriously flawed in design *(19)*. The purpose, risks, and

The Declaration of Helsinki

The internationally recognized doctrine that defined basic human rights in research involving human subjects is the Declaration of Helsinki, adopted in 1964 by the World Medical Assembly and last revised in 2000. The Declaration established that "the interest of science and society must never take precedence over considerations related to the well-being of the subject" (16). The Council for International Organizations of Medical Sciences (CIOMS) issued Proposed International Guidelines for Biomedical Research Involving Human Subjects, which are guidelines for the application, particularly in developing countries, of the principles of the Declaration (17).

benefits of the research should be described to potential respondents in language they can understand, so that they have the information needed to decide whether to participate in the research. Providing this information allows for the *informed consent* of participants. They should be told that they do not have to participate, that they can refuse to answer any question(s), and that they can quit at any time *(20)*. Participant confidentiality should be protected to the extent provided by law. The researcher should not promise absolute confidentiality, if that is a greater degree of confidentiality than the law permits *(11)*. For example, under certain circumstances, confidential information can be subpoenaed by a court of law. The Public Health Service Act of the United States provides additional protections for sensitive data under Sections 308(d) and 301(d).

Confidential research data may be protected from inappropriate or inadvertent disclosure by precautions such as the following:

- Developing a system (i.e., identification [ID] numbers) for storing and tracking questionnaire data without using personal identifiers.

- Keeping all identifying documents or files locked away or password protected and separate from questionnaire data.

- Allowing access to identifiers only to research staff with a legitimate need for it.

- Specifying a time for destroying linkages to identifiers after data retrieval is completed.

TYPES OF QUESTIONNAIRES AND MODES OF ADMINISTRATION

A questionnaire can be administered in a variety of ways, such as in person or over the telephone by an interviewer, or through postal or electronic mail services without the aid of an interviewer. Each mode of administration has potential strengths and weaknesses and necessitates the use of a certain type of questionnaire. Most often, if the study's objectives are clearly defined, its population clearly identified, and its budget and resources clearly understood, then the choice of questionnaire and mode of administration become obvious *(21)*.

In epidemiologic studies, two main types of questionnaires are used: interviewer-administered and self-administered. These two types can be further classified by the manner in which they are administered. Researchers may use different types of questionnaires and methods of administration in the same study in an effort to increase data quality and efficiency of data collection. For example, an interviewer may administer a questionnaire to study participants during their visit to a health care provider, then give them a self-administered questionnaire concerning medication usage to complete at home, where they can access their prescriptions. Researchers may administer a questionnaire over the telephone as an initial eligibility screening tool and then conduct a more detailed in-person interview of eligible respondents.

Computerization is playing an increasingly important role in standardizing interviews, decreasing the time spent on individual interviews, and simplifying coding and data entry. Internet-based surveys already are practical for use in selected groups and show great potential for use in the future as access to and familiarity with computers, e-mail, and the Internet increase *(22)*. In the late 1900s, for example, the number of Internet subscribers in Africa increased from less than 15,000 to over 400,000 *(23)*. As of 2001, in the United States, more than half the population was using the Internet and 45% percent was using e-mail. Internet use is increasing across income, education, age, race, ethnicity, and gender groups, with 2 million new users per month *(24)*.

The following brief overview of the resource-rich literature concerning questionnaire design is based on the work of several authors, including A. E. Bennett, K. Ritchie, Doug R. Berdie, John F. Anderson, Marsha A. Niebuhr, Lu Ann Aday, Ann Bowling, William Nicholls, Reginald P. Baker, Jean Martin, Jennifer L. Kelsey, W. Douglas Thompson, and Alfred S. Evans *(2, 21, 25–28)*.

Interviewer-Administered Questionnaires

Interviewer-administered questionnaires are better for collecting complex information than self-administered ones because interviewers can be trained to elicit appropriate and more complete information through the use of techniques such as standardized probing. An interviewer-administered questionnaire can be designed for use either in person or over the telephone, whichever is more suitable for the particular study. Pencil-and-paper questionnaires have been used traditionally in interviewer-administered interviews, but computer-assisted telephone interviews (CATI) and computer-assisted personal interviews (CAPI) are being used increasingly in the United States and elsewhere, particularly in large national surveys *(26)*.

Whether a questionnaire is administered in person or by telephone, the personal characteristics of interviewers and the training and supervision they receive are critical to collecting accurate and consistent data from respondents *(21)*. Interviewers should be trained and monitored both to uniformly administer the questionnaire and to record the responses in a standard fashion *(2, 21)*. Traditional supervisory monitoring methods include reviewing a portion of paper questionnaires, periodic observation of interviewers while they are conducting interviews, and assessment of tape-recorded interviews. New quality control methods such as analysis of keystroke files from computerized interviews have also been developed. As with traditional methods, the effectiveness of various new quality control methods has not been evaluated in controlled studies, although the value of supervisory quality control is regarded by many investigators as self-evident *(28)*.

In-person interviews provide the interviewer with more control of the interview process. The interviewer can observe the demeanor of the respondent and make note of any apparent confusion or distraction *(2)*. Visual aids such as cards showing response categories and medication photobooks can be used by interviewers as they administer the questionnaire, and interviewers can be trained to take measurements and collect biologic samples, if necessary. Information collected by interviewers may be recorded via pencil-and-paper or laptop computer. With the latter, questions on sensitive topics that respondents may be reluctant to discuss with an interviewer, such as illicit drug use and sexual behavior, data quality may be enhanced by passing the computer to the respondent for direct entry of responses. These and other methods for obtaining high-quality sensitive data continue to be investigated *(13, 28)*.

In-person interviews, however, can be time-consuming and expensive. Interviewers must tactfully deal with participant schedules and often must make multiple attempts to contact and meet with participants *(2)*. Although the best response rates have historically been achieved with in-person interviews *(25)*, recent large, well-funded studies have achieved response rates of 80% or less *(29, 30)*. These results suggest that response rates have dropped and that higher rates may no longer be achievable.

Telephone interviews may be less costly than those administered in person, saving as much as 50% *(31)*. Geographically dispersed populations with widespread residential telephone coverage can be reached more efficiently, without the cost in time and money required to travel interviewers from one respondent to another. Telephone interviews can be readily monitored by supervisors *(26)*, and deviations in interviewing technique can be quickly identified and corrected. In addition, interviewers can safely telephone respondents from undisclosed locations rather than traveling to respondent homes or other meeting places (2). Data from telephone interviews have been shown to be comparable in quality to those from in-person interviews (32). In recent years, touch tone data entry (TTDE) and voice recognition (VR) technologies have opened the door to telephone "interviews" that can be conducted entirely by a computer (28). These technologies may prove important for reducing costs, enhancing accurate reporting of sensitive data, reducing the extent of missing data, and improving response rates for interviews as a whole.

Telephone interviews generally have yielded response rates higher than those of self-administered postal surveys, although somewhat lower than those of in-person interviews (2). The growing use of telephone answering machines and other devices such as "Caller ID" to screen incoming calls may serve to further reduce participation in telephone surveys (26, 33). Study affiliation with a respected organization and the use of introductory letters mailed prior to making telephone contact (26, 27), however, may help combat these influences and improve response rates for telephone interviews.

Information collected in a telephone interview is generally less complex than that collected during an in-person interview. In general, the balance of control in the interview is shifted toward the respondent. Visual aids can be mailed to respondents in advance, but they cannot be administered by the interviewer during the interview, and the interviewer has relatively little control over distractions and influences in the respondent's environment.

One potential problem of telephone interviewing is that significant selection bias may be generated by including only persons with a telephone. Residential telephone coverage varies widely around the world. Apart from country-to-country variation, coverage may differ by region and socioeconomic group within a given country (35). In addition to coverage considerations, telephone sampling has been made more complicated by overlapping area codes, cellular telephones, and increasing numbers of households with multiple telephones and combinations of traditional and cellular telephones.

Self-Administered Questionnaires

Self-administered questionnaires are useful for collecting simple information that is relatively easy for respondents to provide. Without the expenses associated with study interviewers, use of self-administered forms is more economical and practical for collecting data from large numbers of respondents, particularly when dispersed over wide geographic areas. The absence of an interviewer also prevents the introduction of interviewer bias in the data. In addition, evidence suggests that respondents may be more willing to disclose certain kinds of sensitive information when an interviewer is not involved *(35)*. Self-administered questionnaires can be delivered to participants in a group setting, such as a clinic, research facility, or workplace, or individually through the postal service or the Internet. The ability of the researcher to standardize data collection is limited in self-administered interviews, however, regardless of whether or not a staff person is present. No matter how carefully a questionnaire is formatted to facilitate correct interpretation of individual questions and to direct respondents through the appropriate questions in the correct order, respondents are generally free to read the entire interview at the outset and proceed in any way they choose.

Self-administered questionnaires completed in the presence of research staff yield a higher response rate than those delivered via the postal service. The presence of study staff allows for personal contact with respondents, clarifications regarding the study or study materials if needed *(36)*, and some degree of monitoring of the environment in which data are collected. In addition, persons with specific exposures or health conditions of interest, who can be easily identified by the staff who are present, can be targeted and recruited individually to complete the questionnaire. For example, pregnant women with a history of premature delivery could be identified and recruited to complete a questionnaire by clinic staff while waiting for their regular prenatal appointment; an occupational cohort with a common exposure could be identified and gathered together at the workplace to complete individual questionnaires. Although this approach is efficient, it usually is not suitable for studies where sampling is required. In a group setting, the CASI technique can be used, provided a computer lab or other similar facility is available.

Self-administered questionnaires distributed and returned by mail can be rapidly and widely disseminated to a large number of potential respondents to collect simple information on a wide variety of topics. They may be particularly useful for collecting sensitive information that respondents may be reluctant to provide to an interviewer or record in the presence of research staff. Distribution of questionnaires by mail is generally not suitable for collecting complex information because the respondents must read and interpret the questions by themselves without any clarification. Other household members could "help" with the questionnaire, which is usually undesirable. Respondents may review the questions and answer in any order they choose. Although mailed questionnaires are easily disseminated in settings with widespread and dependable postal service, they often initially meet with relatively low response; the occurrence of major societal events may further reduce survey response by increasing the likelihood that unfamiliar or unexpected mail will not be opened (37). Response rates can be increased through the use of follow-up mailings (38, 39), although these can be costly and do not necessarily ensure against bias (40, 41).

Types of questionnaires and modes of administering them are rapidly evolving, largely as a result of advances in telecommunication and computer technology. Social norms, which may influence response rates and accuracy of data, are changing as well. The more researchers know about a variety of technological and other factors in the study population, the better equipped they are to select the most appropriate type of questionnaire for their study. Unfortunately, research concerning the effects of emerging technologies and social factors on questionnaire design and administration is lagging behind the pace at which these changes are occurring (22). Nonetheless, researchers armed with knowledge of study objectives, available resources, and basic characteristics of the study population should not have difficulty choosing the most appropriate type of questionnaire for most epidemiologic studies. Key information presented above is summarized in Figure 4.

BASICS OF QUESTIONNAIRE DESIGN

Answering a question, even a seemingly simple one, requires a number of sequential tasks. A respondent must first interpret the question, then recall the necessary information from memory, next evaluate the relevance of the information and perform any estimates that may be needed, and finally edit and prepare the response for delivery (42). Depending on the characteristics of the question and the respondent, some of these tasks may be more burdensome for the respondent or more likely to result in error than others. In Figure 5, a respondent contemplates his answer to the interviewer's question: "On average, during the years that you smoked, how many cigarettes per day did you smoke?"

Figure 4. Factors to Consider When Selecting the Type of Questionnaire		
	Interviewer-Administered Questionnaire	Self-Administered Questionnaire
Response	Generally higher	Generally lower
Ability to Monitor Data Collection	Easy to limited	Limited to impossible
Interviewer Error	Present	None
Relative Cost	Higher cost	Lower cost
Time in Field	Longer data collection period	Shorter data collection period
Maximum Length	60–90 minutes	30 minutes
Complexity of Questions	Higher complexity	Lower complexity
Use of Visual Aids	Easy	Difficult
Sensitive Topics	Decreased respondent comfort	Increased respondent comfort

When designing a questionnaire, investigators must weigh the questions they would like to ask against the limitations of what most respondents are able and willing to provide. Failure to consider respondent burden when constructing a questionnaire will result in poor quality data *(11)*. The selection and construction of survey questions starts with the list of variables developed by the investigator in the study proposal. The variables, as well as examples of previously used questions and related questionnaires are compiled during the investigator's review of the epidemiologic and medical literature (See Chapter 2: Developing a Research Proposal). Developing table shells as a part of the analysis plan is widely recommended as an efficient method of identifying the variables that will be needed. Table shells are also useful in minimizing the inclusion of unnecessary variables on the list and unnecessary questions in the questionnaire. Once the variables are identified, questionnaire development can proceed.

Figure 5. Thinking About Answers

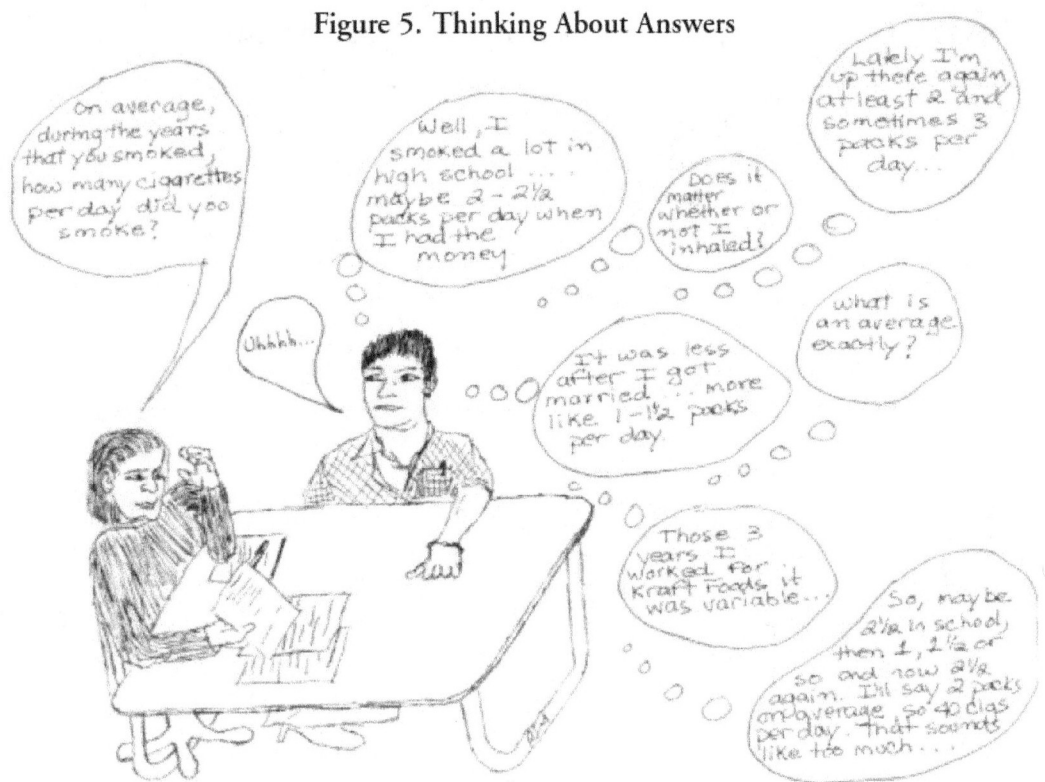

Illustration: Peter J. McDonald, 2001

Validity and Reliability

The concepts of validity and reliability (Chapter 4: Epidemiologic Study Design) are most often used in epidemiologic research to evaluate how well a given question will yield an accurate and precise measure, or the true value, of the phenomenon under study *(3)*. Assessing measurement error in this way is primarily a statistical process and is usually carried out in separate studies designed specifically for that purpose *(43)*. (See *Statistical Assessment of Measurement Error*, p. 67.)

The term *validity* is also used frequently in reference to the inferences that can be drawn from survey data. For example, in a study designed to examine access to routine medical care, asking respondents only for the number of times they have visited a physician in the last month will not provide a valid measure of access to care for those who typically choose to see a nurse practitioner instead of a physician. When designing a questionnaire, investigators must also be attentive to this kind of validity.

Assessment of validity and reliability in the context of questionnaire design involves qualitative as well as quantitative procedures, which are integrated throughout design activities. (See *Pre-Survey Evaluation of the Questions and the Questionnaire*, p. 46.) Extensive research into the question and answer process has identified important characteristics of questions and the way in which they are administered that affect validity and reliability. Study investigators need to be aware of these factors as they design and assess the usefulness of their questions and questionnaires. These factors, or characteristics, are discussed below within the context of the general design objectives stated earlier.

Borrowing Questions from Other Questionnaires

Before embarking on the design of new questions, however, it is important to review the literature and evaluate the utility of similar questions from previous studies. It is common in epidemiology and considered good practice to borrow questions and questionnaires developed by previous investigators whenever possible. When legal, borrowing questions is not only efficient, but improves the comparability of data collection instruments used in different studies and the comparability of findings resulting from these studies *(44, 45)*. Increasingly, scientific journals and health agencies are making available copies of questions and questionnaires that are not copyrighted, e.g., materials developed by the U.S. government *(45–47)*. For example, the Web sites of the CDC's National Center for Chronic Disease Prevention and Health Promotion (www.cdc.gov/nccdphp) and National Center for Health Statistics (www.cdc.gov/nchs) contain the instruments of several national surveys conducted by the U.S. government. These questionnaires and related documentation can be accessed directly and used free of charge. In addition, investigators should feel free to contact authors of published studies to request copies of data collection forms that are otherwise unavailable.

Many of these borrowed instruments have been previously tested for the validity and reliability of the responses they elicit. Such prior assessment is helpful in that it provides information about the quality of data collected previously with these questions, and it may limit additional testing that will be needed for the current study. However, it is important to know the type and purpose of any prior testing, when the testing was conducted, and the characteristics of the population in which the testing occurred, because validity and reliability are tied to these factors *(44)*. Investigators will need to evaluate the circumstances under which previously used questions were tested, determine the applicability of previous results to the current study population and setting, and plan for additional tests as needed. On the basis of these results, investigators should weigh the advantages of borrowing questions and the comparability with previous research this may engender against any limitations of the questions in the current setting, and make informed decisions to keep and use the questions as they are or to make changes to them *(13, 25)*.

Types of Questions

Broadly speaking, survey questions can be formatted in two ways: as open questions, or questions that will accept any information provided by the respondent, and as closed questions, or questions that restrict the respondent to choosing between prespecified responses. A goal for every question included in a questionnaire, regardless of format, is to clearly convey what type of information is being sought *(48)*. In questionnaires designed for epidemiologic study, use of closed questions is commonly maximized to increase question specificity; more specific responses facilitate quantitative analysis and increase the comparability of results across studies *(45)*. Nevertheless, researchers generally agree that each format has strengths and limitations and that use of open, closed, or mixed format questions should be guided by the purpose of the question being asked and the type of information it asks for.

Open questions: Open-ended questions ask respondents to recall or retrieve information without spelling out the possible responses for them. As a result, these questions can be burdensome for respondents, interviewers, and coders, especially if they are complicated and lead to detailed answers. In epidemiology, the open format is typically used to collect simple, factual data, in questions for which many possible responses exist. Demographic data and exposure data, which can be coded directly without loss of information, are well-suited to the open format *(43)*. For example:

Example 1. Open Format Questions

Q1. What is your date of birth? |__|__| |__|__| |__|__|__|__|
                                                month   day   year

Q13. In the *3 months before* you got pregnant, how many cigarettes or packs of cigarettes did you smoke on an average day? (A pack has 20 cigarettes.)

                   ____Cigarettes OR ____ Packs

Adapted from CDC/NCCDPHP/DRH. Pregnancy Risk Assessment Monitoring System (PRAMS). Atlanta; 1987.

Example 2. Open Format Questions of a Sensitive Nature

Q16b. In the *3 months before* you got pregnant, how many times did you drink 5 alcoholic drinks or more in one sitting?

____Times

Adapted from CDC/NCCDPHP/DRH. Pregnancy Risk Assessment Monitoring System (PRAMS). Atlanta; 1987.

In addition, questions about some potentially sensitive topics, such as alcohol use or sexual behavior, may yield more complete or accurate responses in the open format, perhaps because respondents feel more comfortable reporting socially undesirable behavior if no suggestions of normality are implied by prespecified response categories *(11, 45)*.

Another common use of the open format in epidemiology is in the pre-evaluation of questions as a way to identify the range of expected responses and develop the appropriate response categories that will be used in the finalized questionnaire *(21, 48, 49)*.

Closed questions: Closed-ended questions can include dichotomous or multiple choice questions, checklists, and rating scales *(21, 27)*. They are used extensively in self-administered questionnaires and in other questionnaires where complicated or subjective information, such as knowledge or feelings, is being collected *(43)*. Advantages of using specified response categories are that they remind respondents of important experiences they may otherwise have forgotten or been unable to express and, by providing respondents with more information about how to answer the question, they limit the kinds of responses that will be given *(48)*. When collecting information about past experiences in epidemiologic questionnaires, listing the responses of interest in a closed format may yield better information than ask-

Example 3. Closed Format Question		
Did you have any of these problems during your pregnancy? For each item, circle Y (Yes) if you had the problem or circle N (No) if you did not.	No	Yes
a. Labor pains more than 3 weeks before your baby was due (Preterm or early labor)	N	Y
b. High blood pressure (including preeclampsia or toxemia) or retained water (edema)	N	Y
c. Vaginal bleeding	N	Y
d. Problems with the placenta (such as abruptio placentae, placenta previa)	N	Y
e. Severe nausea, vomiting, or dehydration	N	Y
f. High blood sugar (diabetes)	N	Y
g. Kidney or bladder (urinary tract) infection	N	Y
h. Water broke more than 3 weeks before your baby was due (premature rupture of membranes, PROM)	N	Y
i. Cervix had to be sewn shut (incompetent cervix, cerclage)	N	Y
j. You were hurt in a car accident	N	Y
Source: CDC/NCCDPHP/DRH. Pregnancy Risk Assessment Monitoring System (PRAMS). 1987.		

ing a completely open-ended question.

Unspecified response options and options for unknown responses are commonly added to closed questions in epidemiologic surveys. In the next example, investigators have added a category for "Other (specify)" to the response options, in case the respondent feels the specified categories do not adequately describe the place where her prenatal visit occurred. A respondent who was visited by a nurse in her home, for instance, might check the "Other (specify)" option and write in "at my home." A category for "Don't know" has also been added. The availability of this option will increase the accuracy of response overall, since respondents who are not sure of the right answer will choose "Don't know" rather than guess *(48)*. If completeness of the data is more important than accuracy, however, it may be preferable not to offer a "Don't know" response.

Closed questions may lead to increased errors if they suggest an answer that a respondent may not have otherwise provided (e.g., if a respondent thinks an item is familiar when it is not, or if all of the prespecified responses are not read by a respondent in a self-administered questionnaire) *(21)*. In all closed questions, the completeness and number of response options included, the wording and phrasing of each and the order in which they are presented can make critical differences in the quality and usefulness of the data collected *(43, 48)*. To minimize the extent to which these factors influence responses, design and testing of response options should be given the same attention as the design and testing of the questions themselves.

Example 4. Question That Includes Response Categories for "Other" and Unknown

Q10. Where did you go for your first prenatal visit? Please choose one answer and specify the name of the facility. (READ RESPONSES)

❑ 1   Hospital clinic

❑ 2   Health department clinic

❑ 3   Private doctor's office

❑ 4   Birthing center

❑ 5   Community health center

❑ 8   Other (specify) _____

❑ 9   Don't know

Name of facility_____

Design Characteristics of Questions and Their Administration That Influence Measurement

Design Objective 1: Communicate meaning consistently.

The first objective of a well-designed question is that it be interpreted to mean the same thing by all respondents. Since individuals use their life experience to interpret requests for information, study populations that are diverse with respect to ethnicity, age, education, or other cultural factors will interpret and respond to questions differently *(50)*. In most study populations, even basic terms that would seem to carry widely shared meanings can be surprisingly problematic. As a result, investigators must carefully examine the way respondents interpret key words and phrases before questions are finalized. In addition, survey research and experience have shown that the efficiency of the question-naire construction process and the quality of the final product is greatly enhanced if designers avoid certain common pitfalls described below.

Avoid vague and difficult language. In general, investigators can use two approaches to increase the likelihood that respondents will inter-pret terms consistently: 1) build definitions of ambiguous, abstract, or difficult terms into the question itself, and 2) avoid these terms (and their complicated definitions) by asking a series of questions that cover all aspects of what is to be reported and allow investiga-tors to compute the exposure or event for themselves with the data collected. For example, in the relatively simple medical history ques-tion in Example 5, study investigators chose to include definitions of medical terms within the body of the question *(51)*:

Example 5. Defining Medical or Other Terms Within the Question

Q. Before (REFERENCE DATE), did a doctor or other health professional ever tell you that you had phlebitis, pulmonary embolism, or blood clots in your legs or lungs?

In a more complicated and frequently used question about the use of medical care shown in Example 6 *(13)*, however, investigators chose not to define the terms *seen, talked,* or *health professional,* which would have added to the question's complexity.

Example 6. Question Using Broad Undefined Terms

Q1. In the past year, have you seen or talked with a doctor or other health professional about your health?

YES . . . . 1 (Skip to Q4)

NO 2

To ensure that respondents would report telephone consultations and care received from psychiatrists, for example, follow-up questions such as those shown in Example 7 could be added.

Example 7. Follow-up Questions to Probe for More Information

Q2. In the past year, have you talked over the telephone with a doctor or other health professional about your health?

Q3. In the past year, have you seen or talked with a psychiatrist about your health?

Adapted from: Fowler FJ Jr. Improving survey questions: design and evaluation. Thousand Oaks, CA: Sage Publications, Inc.; 1995.

Many types of words may be interpreted in various ways and should be defined or avoided in diverse populations. These include vague terms used to measure frequency of events, such as *usual, average, frequent, regular, occasional, often;* vague descriptive terms, such as *old* or *wealthy;* evaluative terms, such as *good* or *bad;* vague pronouns, such as *you,* that can be interpreted personally or collectively; abbreviations; jargon; colloquialisms; and slang. Difficult or sophisticated terms are also frequently misinterpreted. A key factor in the interpretation of words and phrases is the readability of the text. Investigators should be aware of vocabulary and educational level of the target population and aim to communicate at that level *(21).* In general, the wording of questions should be as straightforward, simple, and specific as possible. In the first question in Example 8, a vague term, *smoke,* and a vague descriptor of frequency, *regularly,* are used; in the second question they are replaced with more specific language:

> **Example 8. Avoiding Ambiguous Terms**
>
> Q1. How old were you when you first began to smoke regularly? (*vague*)
>
> Q2. How old were you when you first smoked one or more cigarettes a day for one month or longer? (*more specific language*)

Another fairly common source of ambiguity is the use of negative phrasing in a question that can have a negative answer *(42)*, or the so-called double negative. In Example 9, a negative response to the first question shown could mean either that the respondent never uses condoms or does use condoms. (A positive response could also be difficult to interpret.) It is best to avoid this kind of problem by eliminating the negative phrasing.

> **Example 9. Avoiding Negative Phrasing**
>
> Q1. Do you never use condoms?
>
> Q2. Have you used condoms one or more times in the past month?

Q1 in Example 9 illustrates an additional ambiguity, i.e., a nonspecific time frame; does *never* mean not even once in your lifetime, never in recent years, or what exactly? If a specific time frame is not specified in the question, respondents will make up their own minds about what time frame is implied and answer the question accordingly. The phrasing shown in Q2 in Example 9 provides for more consistent interpretation. As shown, in Example 10 as well as in several of the previous examples, questions sometimes are framed around a specific reference date *(43, 52)*, such as a diagnosis date, which is written in for each subject before administering the questionnaire. Questions also may be framed around a particular reference event, such as a pregnancy *(53)*.

Example 10. Reference Dates or Events

Q2. Before (*Reference Date*), were you ever diagnosed with breast cancer?

Q3. In the month before you got pregnant with your new baby, how many times a week did you take a multivitamin?

Sometimes the meaning of an entire question is ambiguous because it fails to convey its intent. A question that starts with the word *why* may be particularly prone to this weakness, since it could be asking for a cause, a goal, an enabling factor, or something else *(54)*. In Q1 of Example 11, investigators were interested in gathering diagnostic information, but respondents interpreted the question in a variety of ways and answered accordingly. The intent of the question is clarified in Q2.

Example 11. Avoiding Ambiguous Intent

Q1. Why were you seeing Dr. _____*Name*_____ at _____*Hospital*_____?

(*ambiguous intent*)

Possible responses:
A1a: Because my mother went to him and she liked him.
A1b: Because it is close to where I live.
A1c: Because I wanted to go to the pharmacy there at the same time.

(*ambiguity clarified*)

Q2. What medical condition or problem caused you to see Dr. _____*Name*_____ at _____*Hospital*_____?

Avoid multiple ideas and concepts. Limiting a question to a single idea or concept is also a requirement for consistent interpretation. In Example 12 *(21)*, it is confusing and unnecessary to include the timing of the event, as shown in Q1, since in this case its timing is unimportant; Q2 is a better question.

Example 12. Avoiding Multiple Concepts
(*multiple concepts*)
Q1. Have you had swelling of both ankles or feet in the morning or later in the day?
(*single concept*)
Q2. Can you tell me, have you ever experienced swelling of both ankles or both feet?

The introduction of multiple ideas can also lead to asking two questions in one, or so-called "double-barreled" questions, especially in instances where the connecting words *and* or *or* are used. In a case-control study of malignant melanoma, in which time frame and other parameters of response were set in previous questions, the question shown in Example 13 was included *(55)*:

> **Example 13. Multiple Concepts**
>
> Q1. How many times have you used temporary hair dyes or color rinses?

The question resulted in an unexpected positive finding, but failure to have distinguished between hair dyes and color rinses, which contain different types of chemicals, limited the investigator's ability to interpret the finding *(43)*.

The single concept requirement does not necessarily mean that short questions are better than long ones. Some investigators have found that longer questions, provided they are restricted to simple language and single ideas, may sometimes yield more accurate or complete responses *(11, 45, 56)*. Various mechanisms could explain this finding, if true. For example, a longer question could give respondents more time to recall information needed to answer the question. Question length is a topic that could be explored in questionnaire pretesting and would benefit from further research *(48)*.

Avoid leading questions. It is probably impossible to design a question that is perfectly balanced and neutral. The very fact that a question is asked means that the investigator thinks it is of interest, and that will suggest certain answers to certain respondents *(48)*. It is comparatively easy, however, to consider the relative balance among combinations of words and phrases to determine 1) whether all sides of a question are adequately represented and 2) whether the question is clearly weighted (or loaded) in one direction or another *(26)*, so that obvious problems can be avoided. Leading questions elicit biased responses because they indicate what the answer should be or the investigator's own point of view *(3)*. In Q1 in Example 14, failure to state alternative sides of the question could inadvertently lead respondents, whereas stating the alternatives, as shown in Q2, could minimize bias *(3)*.

Example 14. Avoiding Leading Questions

Q1. Do you prefer being examined by a doctor of your own sex?

Q2. Would you rather be examined by a male or by a female doctor, or doesn't it matter which?

Loaded words or phrases, such as *unfaithful*, *natural*, *interfere*,

---

Example 15. Avoiding Overlapping Response Categories

Q1. What was the worker's compensation claim for?

(*Overlapping*)	(*Mutually Exclusive*)
A. Chronic lung disease	A. Chronic lung disease
B. Injury	B. Ingestion of a poison
C. Poisoning	C. Burn of the skin
D. Burn	D. Other acute injury
E. Other (specify)	E. Other (specify)

---

motherly, *starvation*, and *intelligent* automatically suggest approval or disapproval *(3)*. In the following example, the leading word *banned* is used in Q1, but is replaced with more neutral language and phrasing in Q2:

Example 16. Using Neutral Terms and Language

Q1. Do you think that smoking should be banned in planes?

Q2. Do you think that smoking should be permitted or not permitted in planes?

Source: Armstrong BK, White E. Principles of exposure measurement in epidemiology. Oxford University Press; 1992.

Some leading questions may be harder to recognize than others because they use terms that can be neutral in some contexts and among some groups of people, but highly loaded in other contexts and among other groups. Consider, for instance, such terms as *birth control* and *abortion*. Pretesting of questions that use these kinds of terms may be the only way investigators can determine how they will be interpreted by respondents.

Avoid inadequate and incomplete response categories. Many investigators have explored the ways in which preset response categories in close-ended questions can bias the answers of respondents *(48)*, but the key to conveying consistent meaning to respondents is to offer complete and unambiguous response options. To achieve completeness, investigators must identify and cover all answers respondents are likely to provide; failure to be complete will increase nonresponse and frustrate respondents, whether the questionnaire is self- or interviewer-administered. To avoid ambiguity, investigators must be wary of the same pitfalls described above and be especially attentive to the exclusivity of each response category. Overlapping response options can usually be caught and eliminated during questionnaire testing; nevertheless, errors like those shown in the first set of responses in Example 16 are commonly seen. Since injuries can result from poisonings and burns, respondents with these kinds of claims will be confused about how to answer this question on a self-administered form. Testing might reveal a better set of response options to be something like the second set of responses shown in the example.

Questions involving ages, dates, and intervals of time also commonly fall victim to overlapping response categories. In Example 17, a response of "5 years ago" was coded as category 4 by some interviewers and as category 5 by others, leading to loss of data.

Example 17. Avoiding Overlapping Time Intervals

Q1. When was the last time before (*date*) that you had a breast physical exam?

Never	0
Within 1 year before given date.	1
Within 2 years before given date.	2
Within 3 years before given date.	3
Within 5 years before given date.	4
5 or more years before given date.	5
DK	9

Source: Women's Contraceptive and Reproductive Experiences (CARE) Steering Committee. Women's CARE Study. Atlanta: Public Health Service; NICHD and CDC. 1995.

Design Objective 2: Specify how the question should be answered.

Sometimes the meaning of a question is consistently interpreted, yet the form of the expected answer is not specified and ambiguous. This lack of specificity is especially problematic in open-ended questions that lack preset response options. If the question does not specify how it should be answered, respondents must draw on clues from previous questions, the interviewer, or their own frame of reference. For example, in response to the question below, a variety of reasonable answers could be provided:

Example 18. Lack of Specificity for Answers

Q.   When did you first move to Atlanta, Georgia?

    A1. In 1987.
    A2. When I was 10 years old.
    A3. The summer before I started middle school.

This kind of variation in response will result in increased missing data and increased measurement error, since additional procedures must be conducted to make the data useful. To avoid this problem, the expected form of the answer must be communicated to the respondent. For example, a better question would be one of the following:

Example 19. Providing Specificity for Answers

Q2. In what year did you first move to Atlanta?

Q3. At what age did you first move to Atlanta?

Design Objective 3: Ask for something respondents are able to provide.

Although drawing on a respondent's first-hand experience is generally thought to be the strength of survey research *(13)*, assuming that a respondent is able to provide the answer to any question about his past, present, or future is a mistake. Problems arise because the respondent 1) simply does not have the information, 2) once had the information but cannot recall it, 3) has the information but cannot recall the time period in which the event occurred, or 4) has related information, but cannot provide it in the form the investigator has asked for *(13)*. A critical part of questionnaire design is to make sure that each question can be answered by respondents.

Research has shown that recent and salient events are reported more accurately than more distant and less important ones *(56)*. As a result, relatively routine events, such as visits to the doctor or days lost from work, are best collected only for short periods of time prior to interview (e.g., two weeks) *(13)*, whereas hospital admissions and other unusual events can be more accurately recalled over much longer periods of time *(56)*. For extremely routine events of low saliency, such as dietary practices, one-day recall may be a wise limit. In some studies of routine practices, it has been common to give respondents diaries, asking them to complete and return them at a later date rather than asking them to recall past exposures during the interview *(11)*. Some common strategies to trigger recall of past events and help respondents identify the time period in which they occurred include asking longer questions *(56)*; asking multiple questions about the event *(44, 56)*; using memory aids such as life events calendars *(57–59)*, response cards, photo books, and other, more complex, strategies *(13)*, which are beyond the scope of this chapter. (See p. 32, *Visual Memory Aids*.) In instances where respondents can recall events of interest but cannot provide answers in the form requested, redesign of the question is necessary. One can imagine, for example, that respondents may know exactly where the nearest hospital is located in relation to their home, but may not be able to accurately or reliably report the number of miles between the hospital and their home *(13)*.

Design Objective 4: Ask for something respondents are willing to provide.

Example 20. Establishing a Permissive Attitude

Q. Many people find it difficult to get regular exercise, like jogging, through lack of time. How many times did you go jogging in the past 4 weeks?

Source: Armstrong BK, White E, Saracci R. The design of questionnaires. Principles of exposure measurement in epidemiology. Oxford University Press; 1992.

When respondents feel there is a right or wrong answer to a question, they tend to distort or withhold some responses *(11)*. Their reasons include 1) not wanting to be judged negatively, 2) wanting to answer in a way that is consistent with their own self-image, 3) wanting to answer in a way that is consistent with their answers to previous questions *(12, 26)*, or feeling that a true answer could threaten their well-being (e.g., their marriage, job security, insurance coverage, or standing in the community) *(13)*. Evidence indicates that respondents will underreport embarrassing or socially undesirable events, such as incontinence, abortions *(3)*, and hospitalizations for threatening conditions *(11)*, and overreport events they feel are socially desirable, such as voting *(60)*, owning a library card *(61)*, exercising regularly *(43)*, wearing seat belts, and practicing good personal hygiene *(3)*.

Until questions are actually tested, it is difficult to tell which ones will embarrass or threaten respondents and why. Imagine a respondent who is threatened by a question about age, for example, through fear of personal rejection by the interviewer, fear of mortality, or fear of job-related economic sanctions *(48)*. Because such feelings will influence a respondent's answers, questionnaires should be designed and administered to minimize these reactions *(13)*.

Many design techniques have been described to help reduce distortion in answers to embarrassing or threatening questions *(11, 13, 48, 62)*. The following are believed to be among the most effective and are relatively easy to implement:

- *Ensure that respondents understand the purpose of the question* and why it is important that it be asked. This information can be provided to respondents within the text of the questionnaire, if not within the body of the question itself. Researchers agree that this is the single most important thing an investigator can do to gain the full cooperation of respondents and to minimize distortion in their answers *(48)*.

- *Establish a permissive attitude* by assuring respondents that all responses are acceptable and appropriate, perhaps with an introductory phrase as shown in Example 20, with carefully balanced questions that state all possible answers (see *Avoiding leading questions [3]*), and with generous response categories that encompass even the most extreme behaviors *(48)*.

- *Provide a context for the answer* to reduce the sense that some answers may be interpreted negatively. This can be accomplished through a variety of techniques, including the use of introductory phrases, embedding the question in a series of related, non-threatening questions *(43)* (such as including questions about alcohol consumption among dietary questions or abortion questions among pregnancy history questions), the use of show cards *(3)*, and, in some situations, the deliberate use of leading language to show that the researcher expects and will not be surprised or disappointed by a positive response *(3, 21)*.

- *Restrict the level of detail requested* to that which is essential for analysis. Socially desirable events or exposures are reported more accurately and with less inflation when the length of the reporting period is current or recent rather than usual, and socially undesirable events are reported more accurately when ever or distant events are asked for rather than usual or recent *(13, 43)*. Framing questions about socially undesirable behavior accordingly permits respondents to present themselves in a more positive way currently, while providing the needed information *(13)*.

- *Assure confidentiality.* This involves assuring respondents that many of the issues discussed earlier, including the separation of personal identifiers from data, secure storage of completed questionnaires, restricted access to data of nonstudy personnel, and proper disposal of study instruments, have been and will be carried out *(13)*.

- *Emphasize the importance* of accuracy by having interviewers read statements that emphasize the importance of accuracy to meeting study objectives, asking respondents to commit (verbally or in writing) to providing accurate responses, and training interviewers to selectively reinforce thoughtful answers *(13, 64)*.

- *Reduce or eliminate the role of the interviewer.* This is best accomplished through self-administered questionnaires or by the integration of computer-assisted self-interview (CASI) techniques, touchtone data entry (TDE), voice recognition (VR), randomized response, and other techniques into the personal interview that assure respondent anonymity *(11, 28, 62)*.

Design Objective 5: Administer questions consistently.

In questions presented to respondents in written form or in self-administered questionnaires, all respondents must be able to read the questions, accompanying instructions, and any additional materials provided exactly as written. In questions that are read to respondents by interviewers, interviewers must read the questionnaire and any additional materials provided exactly as written, and any additional information provided by the interviewer (e.g., introductory remarks and answers to respondent questions) must be strictly standardized.

Other Questionnaire Design Factors That Influence Data Quality

The following factors have also been shown to influence the quality of questionnaire data.

Other Standardized Text

General introductory statement. Regardless of the mode of administration, a carefully constructed introductory statement is either read to the respondent by the interviewer or included in the text of the self-administered questionnaire. The primary purpose of this statement is to communicate to the respondent the purpose of the study. Research has demonstrated that when respondents understand why the information they can provide is important, they are more motivated to participate and will work harder to provide complete and accurate data *(64)*. Much of the content of the introductory statement may be presented to respondents in a cover letter at initial contact or during the interview consent process. In addition to conveying the purpose of the study and eliciting respondent cooperation, the introductory statement serves to remind respondents of the confidentiality of the information they provide and to present all of this information in a standardized manner. Other information commonly disclosed in the introduction includes identification of the research organizations and sponsors involved, the interviewer or study director (for mail surveys), the importance of accurate reporting *(65)*, and the fact that participation is voluntary. When respondents are identified on the basis of their disease status (case-control studies) or exposure status (cohort studies), it is common practice for investigators not to mention the specific disease or exposure under study to reduce the possibility that this information will bias response *(43)*.

General instructions. General instructions to respondents for answering questions are a necessity in self-administered questionnaires, but are valuable in interviews as well, since they tell respondents about standard procedures used in the interview process and why they are important (Example 21).

Specific introductions and instructions. Introductory or linking (transitional) statements are often included between subject areas, or modules, to introduce and set the stage for a new topic and to give

---

Example 21. Instructions to Respondents in a Self-Administered Questionnaire

We are asking you to complete this survey so we can learn whether programs that teach students about AIDS and pregnancy are working.

The survey asks questions about preventing AIDS and pregnancy. There are also questions about sexual behavior.

You do not have to answer any questions that make you feel uncomfortable. Your participation is voluntary. It is YOUR CHOICE to answer the questions on this survey. Your grades in school will not be affected by answering this survey.

Your answers will be private. No one at your school will know your answers. It is very important that you answer every question truthfully.

Mark your answers with a #2 pencil. Make dark marks. Erase cleanly any mark you change or stray marks.

Source: Center for AIDS Prevention Studies, ETR Associates. Student health questionnaire. University of California at San Francisco.

---

the respondent in an interview time to refocus. In addition, these kinds of statements can be included within subject areas to break the monotony of a long series of questions (Example 22).

These statements may be phrased somewhat differently in self- and interviewer-administered questionnaires and may need to be kept shorter in the former. In each case, however, they can provide a sense of purpose to questions that might otherwise seem unimportant to the respondent. In addition, they can include specific instructions for answering specific questions. In self-administered questionnaires, this is especially important because serious loss of data can occur from ambiguous or inadequately specified skip patterns or answering procedures that fail to specify, for example, whether a positive response should be indicated by a tick, a circle, or an underline *(13, 36)*.

Interviewer probes and feedback. Instructions as well as any probes and feedback that interviewers may use to communicate with respondents must also be standardized. Ideally, these should be included in the body of the questionnaire, as shown in Example 23. In this example, adapted from a questionnaire developed by Cannell and colleagues, all instructions, probes, and feedback for respondents are italicized, whereas instructions to the interviewer are in uppercase. Probes and feedback instructions may also be provided to interviewers in supplemental question-by-question specifications and training manuals, although this method is not as helpful to interviewers and may lead to increased errors.

Example 22. Specific Introductions, Instructions, and Transitional Statements

K1. (**Introductory Statement**) Now I have some questions about your family history. We are interested in relatives who are living or dead who are related to you by blood.

K3. We will begin with your mother and grand-mothers	K4. Was your (RELATIVE) still living in _____? (REF DATE)	K5. (How old was she?)/ (How old was she when she died?)	K6. Did she ever have cancer before _____? (REF DATE)
Mother	YES 1 NO 2 DK 9	|__|__| AGE	YES 1 NO 2 (K3) DK 9 (K3)
Mother's Mother	"	"	"
Father's Mother	"	"	"

(**Linking/Transitional**) Next, I will be asking similar questions about your sisters, your mother's sisters, and your father's sisters.

(Corresponding table for recording cancer history in <u>sisters</u> and <u>aunts</u> follows.)

Adapted from: *Women's Contraceptive and Reproductive Experiences (CARE) Steering Committee. Women's CARE Study. 1995. Public Health Service: NICHD and CDC.*

Statement of appreciation. Every questionnaire should include a thank you to the respondent for their time and effort *(26)*. Many investigators also include a question asking respondents if they would like to receive a summary of study results when they become available.

Other study documents. In addition to the questionnaires, numerous other documents need to be carefully prepared to ensure that respondents are approached uniformly and receive standardized information about the study. These documents include instruments and methods of initial contact, consent forms, instruction manuals for interviewers, and other documents.

Example 23. Standardized Instructions, Probes, and Feedback

Q1. Let me just mention, to be most accurate, you may need to take your time to think carefully before you answer. (PAUSE) Have you been sick in any way within the last 2 weeks?

IF R SAYS YES:

1a. In what ways were you sick?
1b. Uh-huh, I see. This is the kind of information we want. Were you sick in any other ways within the last 2 weeks?

IF R SAYS NO WITHIN 5 SECONDS:

1c. You answered that quickly. Were you sick in any way at all in the last 2 weeks?
1d. (ANY MENTION) Thanks, this is the kind of information we want.

IF R SAYS NO AFTER 5 SECONDS:

1e. Were you sick in any way at all within the last 2 weeks?
1f. (ANY MENTION) Thanks, this is the kind of information we want.

Adapted from: Cannell CF. Experiments in the improvement of response accuracy. Survey interviewing—theory and techniques. Sydney: George Allen and Unwin, 1985:24-62.

Visual Memory Aids

Memory is not simply a continuous record of the past, but a system of information arrays and event sequences that are stored chronologically and hierarchically in ways that are not well-understood *(66)*. To recall a specific fact or event, a respondent may first need to recall the sequence of events within which the fact is located. The more cues the investigator can provide to help respondents retrieve key information, the better. In addition to cues that may be embedded within questions and any response categories provided, visual aids are commonly employed as memory cues. In personal interviews, for example, response categories are often printed on cards and shown to respondents by interviewers, especially when these categories are numerous. The response card technique can also be used to show respondents a comprehensive list of possible answers for an open-ended question or a list of headings under which all possible responses might fall *(43)*. Photographs, particularly those of specific medications and their packaging, are also believed to enhance recall of past exposures *(43)*. In studies of the effects of exogenous hormones, for instance, it is common practice to prepare photo books containing the names and pictures of all marketed hormones for respondent review *(51)*. Calendars may also be used to record significant life events, and those events can then be used to jog memory of less salient events that would otherwise be more difficult to recall *(42, 51, 58, 59)*. In addition, investigators can ask directly about salient events, such as major illnesses, to improve recall of less salient events, such as medications or procedures the respondent may have been exposed to as a result of those illnesses *(67)*.

Question Order

A respondent's answer to a question is influenced by the questions and answers that precede it in the questionnaire *(68)*. Research indicates that these so-called "order effects," or contextual effects, are caused, in part, by the natural tendency of respondents to generalize to the interview situation expectations they have of speakers in everyday conversation *(10, 66, 69)*.

In particular, respondents will assume that earlier questions may be relevant to later ones. As a result, it is customary for investigators to control order effects by adopting what is called a "funnel approach" *(3, 27, 48)*. Questions are grouped together by subject, starting with the most general and proceeding to the most specific within each group or module. This approach may minimize the burden on respondents as well, because it reduces the amount of time they must spend orienting themselves to new subjects and increases the time available for recall. As much as possible, these question sequences should follow typical patterns of thinking, starting at the present time and going backward to collect an occupational or residential history, for example. The funnel approach often involves "filtering out" respondents to whom the more specific questions do not apply and directing them (or the interviewer) to the next question, or module, that does. It is important to keep these "skips" simple, clear, and, especially in the case of self-administered questionnaires, few in number *(13)*.

In addition to a respondent's expectation that a topic, once covered in the questionnaire, is relevant throughout the interview, most

Example 24.
Problems with Question Order

G3.	G4.	G5.
Before **May 1997** (REFERENCE DATE), did a doctor or other health professional ever tell you that you had any of the following medical conditions?	Looking at the calendar, in what year did a doctor or other health professional **first** tell you that you had (CONDITION)?	Have you ever been hospitalized, had surgery, or been prescribed medication for this condition?
Cancer? YES .... (1) NO .... 2 (G6) DK .... 9 (G6) What type? CODE AS MANY AS APPLY (types of cancer & codes 1-7) COLON .... 6 MELANOMA .... 7 LUNG .... 8 OTHER (SPECIFY) **thyroid**	[ ][ ] [ ][ ] [ ][ ] **8 9** YEAR DIAGNOSED	CANCER CODE FROM G3 [ ][ ] YES .... (1) NO .... 2 DK 9

G6. Before **May 1997** (REFERENCE DATE), did a doctor or other health professional ever tell you that you had a thyroid problem or any condition requiring thyroid medication or treatment?

YES 1
NO .... (2) (SKIP to G13)
DK .... 9 (SKIP to G13)

Source: Women's Contraceptive and Reproductive Experiences (CARE) Steering Committee. Women's CARE Study. 1995. US Public Health Service: NICHD and CDC.

Respondent provided details of thyroid cancer in G3-5, and then answered NO in G6 because she felt she had already provided the information about her cancer and she had no history of other thyroid problems.

respondents will avoid repeating answers to earlier questions and will assume that the investigator is also avoiding redundancy *(10, 12, 69)*. Failure to consider the possible impact of these expectations when making decisions about question order can lead to increased measurement error *(70)*. In example 24, a respondent reports details of her thyroid cancer diagnosis in QG3–5 at the end of a series of medical history questions; in QG6, however, the same respondent answers "no" to a filter question about a history of thyroid disease. This results in a skip to Q13 and failure to collect any information about thyroid medication and radiation that would have been collected in QG7–QG12. After having observed this error several times, study investigators realized that question order was to blame:

respondents were answering "no" to QG6 because, having just told the interviewer about their thyroid cancer, they believed the interviewer would not ask about the same disease again.

Important questions that are easy to answer, but nonthreatening, are usually placed at the beginning of the questionnaire so as not to be affected by earlier questions and answers and any context they may have established. Demographic questions, which are generally of low interest and some of which can be threatening to respondents, should be saved for the end of the questionnaire and ordered so as not to leave the respondent feeling uncomfortable when the interview/questionnaire is completed *(36)*. If study eligibility hinges on one of these questions, religion or race, for example, so that it must be asked in the beginning of the interview, it is helpful to add text explaining why it is important *(43)*. Questions about behavior should precede questions about knowledge or attitudes, since behavior does not always reflect knowledge, and respondents may strive for consistency between the two. The desire to be consistent and even-handed, another characteristic of speakers in everyday conversation, can affect responses throughout the questionnaire *(48)*.

At the end of a questionnaire, it is always a good idea to ask the respondent for comments and feedback, and to allow enough space for verbatim answers to be fully recorded. A typical request for comments, immediately following a thank-you statement, is shown in Example 25.

Question order clearly needs to be considered when borrowing questions from previously designed questionnaires, especially if investigators intend to compare results between the two surveys. If an entire module is borrowed, additional questions on the same topic should be placed at the end of the module or at the end of the form so as not to disturb the context of the earlier questions *(43)*. Unfortunately, strategies to control order effects may have little bearing on self-administered questionnaires, especially those sent through the mail, since respondents are free to read and answer questions in any order they please.

Formatting, Layout, and Related Coding Considerations

A questionnaire should be formatted so as to be as easy to follow as possible. In self-administered forms this is necessary because not all respondents are motivated to take additional time or their reading skills may not be strong. Interviewers can benefit from carefully formatted forms as well because the less attention they have to give to following the form, the more they can focus on administering to the

---

Example 25. Statement of Appreciation; Additional Comments

Thank you for taking time to answer these questions. Please use this space for any additional comments you would like to make about the health of mothers and babies.

(Provide large space that will be adequate for written comments)

Adapted from CDC/NCCDPHP/DRH. Pregnancy Risk Assessment Monitoring System (PRAMS). 1987.

---

respondent. As a secondary benefit, careful formatting can ease and reduce error in the subsequent preparation and processing of data. Certain formatting conventions for text, response categories, and overall layout have been shown to enhance data quality and, as a result, are commonly used by survey designers *(13, 27, 43)*.

Conventions for text. Questions should be printed in large font and lowercase typeface; in populations using self-administered questionnaires where vision problems may be prevalent (e.g., the elderly), extra-large typeface may be called for. Question text should be easily distinguished from any printed instructions to the interviewer or respondent; this is especially important on interviewer-administered forms, where it is important to avoid interviewer confusion (and the impression of interviewer confusion) as much as possible. Similarly, skips should be clearly indicated, usually in boldface type, and placed immediately after the answer or response code *(43)*. Examples 26 and 27, from personal interview forms, illustrate these conventions.

As illustrated in Example 28, taken from an interviewer-administered questionnaire *(51)*, conventions are also needed to indicate word choices and substitutions that interviewers must occasionally make, as well as the standardized probes and feedback shown earlier in Example 23.

Example 26. Formatting a Question in an Interviewer-Administered Questionnaire

725.   Have you ever asked a partner to use a condom?

1. YES
2. NO --> GO TO Q727
8. DON'T REMEMBER --> GO TO Q727

727.   If your partner/husband would want to use a condom when having sex with you, would you feel: (READ A-G)

	AGREE	DISAGREE	DK
A. Embarrassed?	1	2	8
B. Angry?	1	2	8
C. Safe from getting pregnant?	1	2	8
D. Safe from getting HIV?	1	2	8
E. Like you had done something wrong?	1	2	8
F. Safe from getting STD?	1	2	8
G. Suspicious that he may sleep around?	1	2	8

Source: Serbanescu F, Morris L, Marin M. Reproductive Health Survey: Romania, 1999. 2001. Atlanta GA; Romanian Association of Public Health and Health Management (ARAPMA); Division of Reproductive Health, Centers for Disease Control and Prevention; US Agency for International Development (USAID); United Nations Population Fund (UNFPA); United Nations Children's Fund (UNICEF).

Example 27. Conventions for Text

2.   In what country were you born?
   ❑ 1   Mexico
   ❑ 7   Other_____ (SKIP to 4)
            (NAME of COUNTRY)

3.   In what state were you born?   _____
                                            (NAME of STATE)

4.   How long have you lived in Mexico?

   ❑ 1   less than 6 mo.
   ❑ 2   6 mo.–less than 1 year
   ❑ 3   1–5 years
   ❑ 4   More than 5 years

Conventions for formatting and recording responses. To enable direct input of data from the questionnaire, closed questions should be precoded, and open questions on interviewer-administered forms should include codes for all anticipated responses. Numerical codes

	G14. Please tell me the name of the medication you (first/next) took at least once a week for one month or longer?	G15. When did you start taking (MEDICATION) regularly?
Example 28. Standardized Word Substitutions and Other Interview Conventions		
1ST MED	_____ NAME |__| CODE	|__|__|/|__|__| MONTH/YEAR
2ND MED	_____ NAME |__| CODE	|__|__|/|__|__| MONTH/YEAR

(table continues 3rd, 4th, etc.)

(WHEN REPEATING G14 ELUCIDATES NO FURTHER MEDS, PROBE TO COMPLETE)	*"Are there any others?"*	RECORD ADDITIONAL MEDICATIONS IN TABLE OR CONTINUATION BOOK AS NEEDED

Source: Women's Contraceptive and Reproductive Experiences (CARE) Steering Committee. Women's CARE Study. 1995. US Public Health Service: NICHD and CDC.

are favored over letter codes because they lead to fewer problems in data processing and analysis, and allow for more unique codes than do the 26 letters. It is important to follow a consistent pattern in assigning code numbers to comparable response categories, using '1' for YES, '2' for NO, and '9' for UNKNOWN, for example, and to assign separate codes for unknowns, refusals, and missing information. Data quality is also served by directing respondents and interviewers to record responses in a consistent manner, circling the coded number, for example, or checking or ticking the response category that applies. See Example 29.

Vertical answer formats for precoded responses have been shown to be less confusing to respondents, interviewers, and data entry personnel than are horizontal layouts *(26, 43)* (Example 30).

Most authors advise aligning response codes along the right-hand

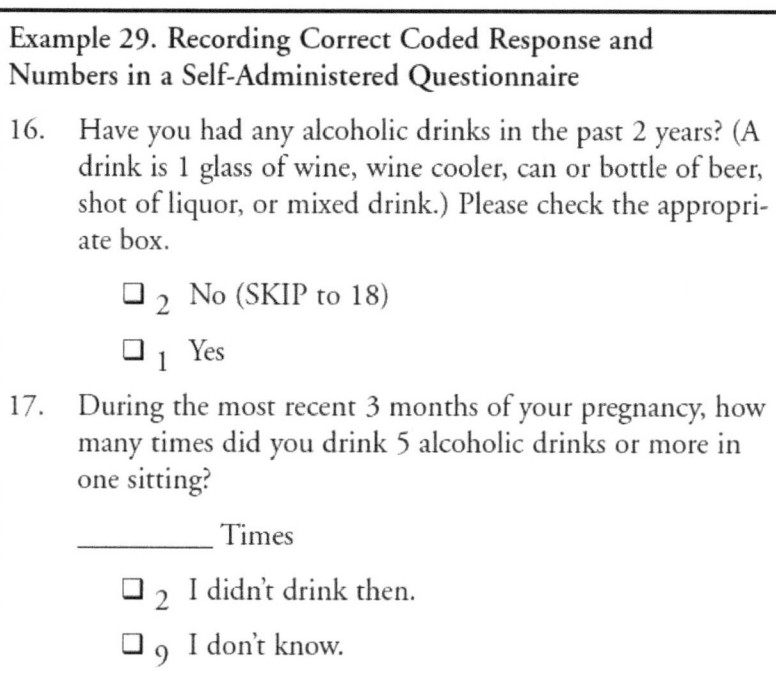

Example 29. Recording Correct Coded Response and Numbers in a Self-Administered Questionnaire

16. Have you had any alcoholic drinks in the past 2 years? (A drink is 1 glass of wine, wine cooler, can or bottle of beer, shot of liquor, or mixed drink.) Please check the appropriate box.

   ❑ 2   No (SKIP to 18)

   ❑ 1   Yes

17. During the most recent 3 months of your pregnancy, how many times did you drink 5 alcoholic drinks or more in one sitting?

   _____ Times

   ❑ 2   I didn't drink then.

   ❑ 9   I don't know.

margin of the questionnaire on telephone or personal interview forms for ease of interviewer recording and data entry *(26, 43)*. On self-administered forms, however, where ease and accuracy of respondent recording is primary, aligning codes to the left of the response categories and in line vertically with codes for questions that precede and follow, is advised *(71)*. See Examples 31 and 32.

For open questions, and other (specify) responses, spaces or boxes should be provided, and the desired units of measurement for open as well as closed questions should always be specified (Example 33).

When respondents are asked to indicate more than one response to a question, recorded answers are easier to interpret if respondents are

---

Example 30. Vertical and Horizontal Answer Formats

17b. During the *most recent 3 months* of your pregnancy, how many times did you drink 5 alcoholic drinks or more in one sitting?

_____ Times

☐ 2 I didn't drink then.

☐ 9 I don't know.

17b. During the *most recent 3 months* of your pregnancy, how many times did you drink 5 alcoholic drinks or more in one sitting?

_____ Times   ☐   I didn't drink then.   ☐   I don't know.

Example 31. Formatting Conventions in an Interviewer-Administered Questionnaire

Q10. Where did you go for your first prenatal visit? Please choose one answer and specify the name of the facility. (READ RESPONSES)

HOSPITAL CLINIC	1
HEALTH DEPARTMENT CLINIC	2
PRIVATE DOCTOR'S OFFICE	3
BIRTHING CENTER	4
COMMUNITY HEALTH CENTER	5
OTHER (SPECIFY) _____	8
DON'T KNOW	9

Name of facility_____

Adapted from: Non-Respondent Questionnaire (NRQ) Women's Contraceptive and Reproductive Experiences (CARE) Steering Committee. Women's CARE Study. 1995. US Public Health Service: NICHD and CDC.

Example 32. Formatting Conventions in a Self-Administered Questionnaire

C7. What is your menstrual status?

1..........Still having periods, or pregnant, or nursing

2..........Possibly beginning menopause, or going through menopause or the change of life

3..........Periods stopped by themselves or natural menopause

4..........Periods stopped by surgery removing uterus (womb) or both ovaries

5........Other (Specify)

Adapted from: Non-Respondent Questionnaire (NRQ) Women's Contraceptive and Reproductive Experiences (CARE) Steering Committee. Women's CARE Study. 1995. US Public Health Service: NICHD and CDC.

Example 33. Formatting to Record Units of Measurement

a. How old were you when you first used birth control pills?

|__|__| (age)

b. How many years altogether in your lifetime have you used birth control pills?

|__|__|(#years)

Adapted from: Non-Respondent Questionnaire (NRQ) Women's Contraceptive and Reproductive Experiences (CARE) Steering Committee. Women's CARE Study. 1995. US Public Health Service: NICHD and CDC.

---

forced to choose between Yes and No for each possible response than if they are asked to indicate only those that apply, as shown in Example 34.

When a series of questions is to be repeated for multiple conditions or exposures, such as all places of residence or all occupations, it is simpler, cleaner, and space-saving to use a matrix format, rather than to format each question for each condition separately *(43, 71)*. Similarly, when a question or series of questions has the same set of

---

Example 34. Formatting Questions That Permit More Than One Response

During any of your prenatal care visits, did a doctor, nurse, or other health care worker talk with you about any of the things listed below? **For each thing, please circle Y (Yes) if someone talked with you about it or N (No) if no one talked with you about it.**

		No	Yes
a.	How smoking during pregnancy could affect your baby	N	Y
b.	Breastfeeding your baby	N	Y
c.	How drinking alcohol during pregnancy could affect your baby	N	Y
d.	Using a seat belt during your pregnancy	N	Y
e.	Birth control methods to use after your pregnancy	N	Y
f.	Medicines that are safe to take during your pregnancy	N	Y
g.	How using illegal drugs could affect your baby	N	Y
h.	Doing tests to screen for birth defects or diseases that run in your family	N	Y
i.	What to do if your labor starts early	N	Y
j.	Getting your blood tested for HIV (the virus that causes AIDS)	N	Y
k.	Physical abuse to women by their husbands or partners	N	Y

Source: Georgia Division of Public Health. Georgia Pregnancy Risk Assessment Monitoring System (PRAMS). 1996.

---

response categories or the same skip pattern, it is preferable to use a column format (e.g., the Yes/No responses in Example 34) *(26)*.

Conventions for overall layout and appearance. Questionnaires that will be seen by respondents should be attractive. Colored covers or subsections, for example, can be effective attention-getters, and many covers include an eye-catching illustration or study logo. In addition to having visual appeal, the study logo, if one is used, and the study name should be carefully selected so as not to offend respondents in any way. Paper and pencil forms are best put in booklets to ease reading and page turning and to avoid page loss *(26)*. The organizations conducting and sponsoring the work should be listed on or inside the front cover, and other key information,

---

Example 35. Questionnaire Cover

Georgia

Pregnancy

Risk

Assessment

Monitoring

System

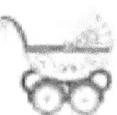
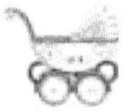
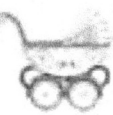

A Survey of the Health of Mothers and Babies

Thank you for your help!

For more information, please call:
Catherine Rohweder
PRAMS Coordinator
1-800-743-7265

Georgia Department of Human Resources
Two Peachtree St., NW, Suite 3513
Atlanta GA 30303

Source: Georgia Division of Public Health. Georgia Pregnancy Risk Assessment Monitoring System (PRAMS). 1996.

---

such as respondent ID and interview date, is also often recorded on the cover. A good cover accomplishes all of this without looking crowded. (See Example 35.)

On interviewer-administered forms, the starting time and ending time of the interview are usually recorded on the first and last pages, respectively. (See Example 36.)

On each page of the questionnaire, ample white space should be pre-

---

Example 36. Recording Elapsed Time of Interview

Page 1

TIME BEGAN: |__|__| : |__|__| AM 1
PM 2

Page 91

TIME ENDED: |__|__| : |__|__| AM 1
PM 2

Source: *Women's Contraceptive and Reproductive Experiences (CARE) Steering Committee. Women's CARE Study. 1995. US Public Health Service: NICHD and CDC.*

---

served, both to avoid the appearance of busyness and to leave room for interviewers to write uncluttered, explanatory notes in the margins; the respondent ID should be recorded or stamped on each. Every question and sub-question should be numbered, and none should ever be split between two pages.

Translation

When studies are conducted internationally or among diverse cultural groups whose members speak different native languages, it is often necessary to translate and administer the questionnaire in two or more languages *(72)*. Translation is a complicated, additional step in questionnaire development that requires careful planning and attention to enhance rather than detract from the quality of data collected *(73, 74)*.

One approach to questionnaire translation that has been recommended by several authors *(43, 75)* is a four-stage process that includes the following: 1) a preliminary translation, 2) evaluation of the preliminary translation, 3) testing for cross-language and cross-cultural equivalence between the translated and original versions, and 4) assessment of validity and reliability of the translated version. The preliminary translation of the questionnaire from the original language into the second should be carried out by a person who is fluent in both languages and well-informed about the objective of the study and the intent of each question. Ideally, a preliminary translator should be as familiar as possible with the culture of the target population as well.

Once the preliminary translation and evaluation are complete, it should be back-translated to the original language by someone with bilingual and bicultural expertise who has not seen the original language version of the questionnaire. Discrepancies must be examined and the translated questions must be redrafted and back-translated again if necessary. This procedure of translation and back-translation may require several iterations until the translated version is satisfactory. New translators and evaluators should be used at each iteration, if possible. In addition to back-translating, bilingual experts can be helpful in examining the translated version and comparing it to the original for content, meaning, and clarity. Once the preliminary translation is complete, the translated questionnaire is tested for cross-language equivalency by administering both versions to bilingual and bicultural respondents and comparing the two sets of responses. Half of the subjects are given the original language version to complete first while half are given the translated version first. Testing for equivalency in this manner is important because back-translation cannot pick up certain kinds of problems (e.g., poor translation that is hidden by compensation skills of good interpreters). Strong correlation between the responses in the two versions of the questionnaire is indicative of cross-language equivalence. The final stage of the translation process, which involves the assessment of validity and reliability, should follow the same pre-survey evaluation procedures as are described for the original version of the questionnaire. (See Pre-Survey Evaluation of the Questions and the Questionnaire, p. 46.) Each translated version of the questionnaire must be assessed separately, because language equivalency does not ensure cultural equivalency, and it is likely that cultural differences between respondents using the translated and original versions of the questionnaire will lead to different interpretations and responses to questions. When limited resources prevent such a carefully planned translation, particularly in instances where respondents are few but vital to the study, less structured and systematic alternatives can be used, such as simultaneous interpretation provided by bilingual interviewers or interpreters. The lack of standardization in these techniques, however, can easily introduce bias into the data *(73)*.

PRE-SURVEY EVALUATION OF THE QUESTIONS AND THE QUESTIONNAIRE

Attention to the design objectives and other considerations described earlier will greatly facilitate the process of constructing a valid questionnaire. The instrument that results, however, is merely a draft. Unfortunately, most investigators spend insufficient time and resources on the important and cost-effective next step of evaluating and testing their drafted questions prior to fielding their questionnaire *(13)*. In part, this may be due to misconceptions about the time and resources required *(13)* and the fact that the best methods of pre-survey evaluation are still being identified *(76)*. Nonetheless, evaluation research has shown that certain relatively simple techniques can be extremely beneficial. These techniques incorporate cognitive and interactional perspectives as well as traditional methods of assessment and include feedback from interviewers and respondents as well as experts and researchers *(13, 45, 48)*. One approach to these methods is to apply them sequentially in phases as described below. The discussion that follows contains an ordered selection of recommended procedures. Readers will need to consult additional sources for more complete information *(13, 45, 48, 66, 76, 77)*.

Phase I: Review by Researchers and Experts

Once the questionnaire has been drafted, it is customary to solicit review and feedback from colleagues and experts who are knowledgeable in the field of study and survey design. This procedure addresses the relevance (or "face validity") and completeness (or "content validity") of the instrument, as well as the meaning of individual questions. Reviewers try to determine whether the questionnaire will measure what it is supposed to measure, whether the right types of information will be captured, and whether the questions will yield accurate answers *(21, 36, 66)*. As a complement to this review, it is helpful for investigators to administer the questionnaire to themselves and a number of willing colleagues, friends, or family members; if the form is designed to be self-administered, a few of these individuals should complete it. These activities can uncover major design problems, which can then be corrected by the investigator.

Phase IIA: Focus Group Discussion with Respondents

These detailed group discussions are geared toward general respondent comprehension of key or problematic questions within the questionnaire *(13, 48, 66)*. Their purpose is to acquaint the researcher with the diversity of experience and perception that may exist in the study target population and to suggest changes to the questions that may be needed to ensure consistent interpretation across that diversity. Focus group discussions, which are typically 1 to 2 hours in length, can yield tremendous amounts of helpful information at relatively low cost. Because results can be diffuse, however, researchers should try to set clear objectives for these discussions. In particular, key recall and reporting tasks and key vocabulary should be identified by investigators beforehand and used to help guide decisions about the composition and number of focus groups that will be needed *(13)*.

Individuals from diverse sociocultural backgrounds, who represent the full range of respondents in the target population, are usually selected by investigators to serve as focus group members. Homogeneous groups may be preferred, however, to address topics that may be difficult to discuss candidly in heterogeneous surroundings (e.g., sexual practices or religious beliefs) *(27)*. Different things can be learned from differently composed focus groups *(13)*. Most investigators report that groups of 5 to 12 members work best.

Focus group discussion centers around whether the selected questions and the words used in them 1) appropriately cover what investigators want the respondents to describe, 2) convey consistent meaning, and 3) pose tasks that respondents are able and willing to perform *(13)*. For example, if questions about early menstrual cycle regularity are being examined, the interviewer may start by asking the group to talk about what "menstrual regularity" and other terms used in the questions mean to them. How accurately and how easily members can recall details of their menstrual cycles in their teenage years should also be discussed, as well as any hesitation or discomfort members may feel about discussing the subject. When problems in the structure, content, or vocabulary of the questions are identified, the group should be encouraged to propose solutions. To expedite the evaluation process and to reach sound conclusions, it is important to carefully document the interactions among the group members. Having a staff member other than the interviewer take notes, and tape-recording or videotaping the session have been suggested as ways to record discussion for better decision-making *(13)*.

Phase IIB: Intensive Interviews with Individual Respondents

These so-called "laboratory" or "cognitive" interviews have been developed by cognitive psychologists and often take place in a laboratory setting where they can be observed by cognitive specialists *(76, 77)*. These interviews are used in pre-survey evaluation to assess the errors that may be introduced as respondents interpret specific questions, recall necessary information, perform judgments, and edit their answers. Different from focus group interviews, which are conducted in group format and provide general feedback on the adequacy of question wording, these interviews are conducted one to one and incorporate strategies that allow investigators to delve much more deeply into what respondents are thinking as they process and answer a question. Investigators should select the same sorts of individuals for these interviews as they do for focus groups, those who will reflect the full range of diversity found in the study population.

If the study is large and sufficient funds are available, it may be optimal to conduct these interviews in cognitive laboratories, but study interviewers, investigators, and other study staff can learn to perform these techniques *(13)*. Even so, individual interviews are more expensive than focus group discussions, since only one respondent is interviewed at a time. All procedures and interactions should be observed and recorded or videotaped so that problems can be detected and flagged for editing and correction *(13, 43)*.

One of the most commonly used intensive interview strategies, and perhaps the one most easily adopted in settings outside of a cognitive laboratory, is the "double interview" *(48)*. In a double interview, the researcher first asks and the respondent answers a series of questions from the questionnaire; then the researcher asks the respondent a series of additional questions to explore how the respondent arrived at the initial answers. These follow-up questions vary, depending on the content of and tasks involved in the initial questions. Respondents may be asked to paraphrase questions or define terms used in the questions, to identify any confusion about the appropriate answers, to describe the degree of confidence they have in the accuracy of their answers, and to elaborate on the process they used to perform any calculations or estimates that may have been called for *(13)*. A double interview may be conducted in person or over the telephone. Example 37 shows a hypothetical example of the double interview technique.

Like focus group discussions, intensive interviews may last up to 2 hours, but typically cover only 15–20 minutes of the questionnaire

---

Example 37. Double Interview Dialog

The interviewer reads the following introduction and questions from the questionnaire to the respondent:

These questions are about some events that may have happened during your most recent pregnancy. Please circle "YES" or "NO" to each of them.

1. Did your husband or partner threaten you or make you feel unsafe in some way? YES NO

2. Were you frightened for the safety of yourself or your family because of the anger or threats of your husband or partner? YES NO

3. Did your husband or partner try to control your daily activities, for example, control who you could talk to or where you could go? YES NO

4. Did your husband or partner force you to take part in any sexual activity when you did not want to (including touch that made you uncomfortable)? YES NO

Next, the interviewer reads the following introduction and follow-up questions to the respondent to explore how he/she answered the previous questions:

Now I'm going to ask you some additional questions about how you answered each of those questions. Starting with the first one, "Did your husband or partner threaten you or make you feel unsafe in some way?":

1. What does *feel unsafe* mean to you?

2. In what ways, if any, does threaten mean something different?

3. Tell me, what did you take into consideration to answer "YES" or "NO" to this question about feeling unsafe or threatened?

Thinking about the question, "Were you frightened for the safety of yourself or your family because of the anger or threats of your husband or partner?":

4. What does *frightened* mean to you?

5. What does *anger* mean to you?

6. . . .

---

due to the added time required for the follow-up questions *(13)*. For additional examples of this and other intensive interview strategies, readers should explore the cognitive psychology and survey literature *(13, 48, 76, 77)*.

Phase II techniques can be used to test self-administered as well as interviewer-administered questions. When using focus groups or intensive interviews to evaluate self-administered questions, it is a good idea to give each respondent a copy of the questions and response categories to read, but to administer the follow-up interview questions and procedures orally. In this way, the cognitive question-answer processes are easier to observe and assess *(13)*. Cognitive interviews are particularly important when applied to self-administered questions because of the lack of interviewer feedback and difficulty in getting respondent feedback during the pretest (see Phase III: Field Pretest) of the questionnaire.

The Phase I and Phase II techniques described so far involve feedback from researchers, experts, and respondents, but not the interviewers and other staff who collect and prepare the data for analysis. These techniques are particularly concerned with the respondent's interpretation of specific questions and how able and willing the respondent is to give accurate answers to those questions. As a result, they reveal information that is ordinarily not apparent to interviewers or respondents during the course of a more typical interview *(45)*. They do not aim to test the entire questionnaire, to examine tabulated data, or assess other procedures used in the data collection process, including respondent contact, interview administration, or data preparation. These objectives fall to the "field pretest" or "pilot test," the final phase of pre-survey evaluation.

Phase III: Field Pretest

The emphasis in field pretesting is to evaluate the complete questionnaire and all procedures related to its administration and the preparation of its data for analysis. Investigators may continue to evaluate the wording and form of questions in the pretest, but they are also interested in some quantitative review of responses to closed questions; the adequacy of rough codes for open questions; the frequency of item nonresponse; the flow of the questionnaire overall, including transitions between sections and skips; the length of the questionnaire; the level of respondent interest and attention; the adequacy of editing, coding, and data-entry procedures; the adequacy of respondent contact procedures; and the completeness of question-by-question specifications for interviewers and other manuals for other study personnel *(45)*. Pretesting is an iterative process, so it is difficult to predict exactly how many pretests should be conducted, although a minimum of two has been suggested *(13, 45)*. Ideally, investigators conduct an initial pretest, identify problems in the instrument or procedures, make needed modifications, and then pretest again; if additional changes are necessary, additional pretests are conducted.

Unlike earlier evaluation activities, it is important that each pretest be conducted among a representative sample of the target population under circumstances that nearly replicate the way data will be collected once the study is under way. This includes utilization of study interviewers, coders, editors, data entry staff, and other study personnel whenever possible. In general, the larger the sample, the more informative the results will be. Investigators experienced in pretest methodology (13, 45) advise that a minimum of 25–75 questionnaires and 5 or more per interviewer per pretest are needed to code and tally the marginal frequencies of response data and examine the variation in response. This examination can reveal gross problems in the questions or response categories themselves, or in the rough codes for open questions, skip patterns, and other major problems with instruments and procedures. Distinguishing between a faulty questionnaire or procedure and respondent idiosyncrasy can be difficult, however, when such small pretest sample sizes are used. Researchers must weigh study objectives and available resources against their own judgment and experience and that of others as they plan for pretest evaluation.

In addition to pretest questionnaire data, another important source of information about problems in the study instruments and procedures is the study personnel involved in the pretest. In interviewer-administered surveys, interviewer feedback is essential. Study interviewers should conduct the pretest interviews and should be required to follow and apply all standardized data collection procedures developed for the study. After the interviews, it is customary for investigators to conduct oral debriefings or request written reports from interviewers, which document the problems encountered during the pretest interviews (45). In practice, however, it is not possible for an interviewer to both conduct the interview according to protocol and, at the same time, objectively monitor the entire interview process for problems. Aside from the difficulty of doing two jobs well at once, an interviewer's perceptions about an activity in which he or she has an active role cannot be objective. A further complication to interviewer reporting occurs when interviewers are debriefed in groups rather than individually, where they may speak more openly. These issues are worrisome because the pretest is the only opportunity the researcher has to identify problems with the questionnaire and procedures as a whole (45). As a result, several techniques have been developed to enhance the value of pretesting, including 1) systematic methods to record interviewer and respondent behavior during the interview, 2) intense and systematic data collection from interviewers after the interview, and 3) systematic probing of respondents after the interview *(13, 45)*. In addition, a thorough and complete pretest will involve systematic review of all data processing procedures, including editing, coding, and data entry, as well as interviews with staff who conduct these procedures. All of these techniques, discussed below, apply to interview-administered questionnaires, whereas only the third and final technique applies to self-administered questionnaires.

Observation of interviewer and respondent interaction

Methods to pretest personal or telephone questionnaires should include objective observation of interviewer and respondent behavior and detailed coding of that behavior. Coding forms can be developed that allow observers to record the frequency and type of interviewer and respondent behavior that occurs at each question *(13, 78, 79)*. Example 38 shows the behavior codes and form used to monitor and evaluate interviewer performance throughout one large case-control study.

During data collection, such a form is useful in identifying interviewers who do not follow standard protocol. When used during pretesting, however, questions that are problematic for interviewers or that require excessive probing and clarification can be easily identified and modified to better meet the objectives of good question design before the questionnaire is fielded *(80)*. To facilitate evaluation of pretest interview observations, data can be compiled onto one table, as shown for a pretest sample size of 25 in Example 39.

The greater the number of deviations noted, the more likely that a problem is present. An arbitrary error rate cut point of 15% or higher is used by some investigators to flag questions that warrant further evaluation *(13, 79)*. In Example 39, questions A1A, A2, A4, and A5 all appear to pose problems to interviewers, respondents, or both. When the nature of the problem can be easily identified, researchers should propose and implement solutions so that questions found difficult to read are altered, terms found difficult to understand are avoided or defined succinctly, and questions classified as "interrupted" or requiring repetition, probing, or clarification are modified accordingly. When the problem is not so obvious, researchers may return to Phase II techniques to find a solution. Questions associated with additional interaction between the respondent and interviewer are less standardized in the way they are administered and more vulnerable to bias. As a result, good question design strives to minimize these questions.

Example 38. Interview Observation Form	

READING QUESTION

11 READS QX EXACTLY AS WRITTEN

12 APPROP PACE AND PAUSES

13 SPEAKS CLEARLY W/ APPROP EMPHASIS

21 READS QX MAKING MINOR CHANGES, NOT CHANGING THE MEANING OF THE QUESTION

22 ALTERS OR OMITS WORDING AND/OR PHRASES, CHANGING THE MEANING OF THE QUESTION

23 FAILS TO READ A QX OR INTRODUCTION

24 MISSES A SKIP PATTERN

25 FAST/SLOW PACE, INAPPROP OR LACK OF APPROP PAUSE

26 DOES NOT SPEAK CLEARLY/LACKS APPROP EMPHASIS

PROBING

31 PROBE IS NEUTRAL AND APPROPRIATE

32 APPROP USE OF EXPECTANT PAUSE

33 REPEATS QX EXACTLY AS WRITTEN

41 FAILS TO PROBE WHEN NECESSARY OR PROBES WHEN NOT NECESSARY

42 PROBE IS DIRECTIVE AND/OR INAPPROPRIATE

43 FAILS TO USE EXPECTANT PAUSE

44 REPEATS QX WITH MINOR CHANGES, NOT CHANGING THE MEANING OF THE QUESTION

45 REPEATS QX ALTERS OR OMITS WORDING, CANGING THE MEANING OF THE QUESTION

OTHER INTERVIEWER BEHAVIORS (NON RECORDING)

51 APPROP INTRO OR EXIT REMARKS

52 HANDLES DISTRACTION APPROP

53 ANSWERS RESPONDENT'S QX APPROPRIATELY

54 OFFERS APPROPRIATE FEEDBACK

61 INTERRUPTS RESPONDENT

62 OFFERS PERSONAL VIEWPOINT

63 ENGAGES IN EXTRANEOUS CONVERSATION

64 FAILS TO APPEAR FOCUSED AND INTERESTED, MAINTAIN EYE CONTACT

65 OFFERS INAPPROPRIATE FEEDBACK OR ANSWERS RESPONDENT'S QUESTIONS INAPPROPRIATELY

CAL-, SHCARDS-, AND PHOTOBK-ASSOCIATED BEHAVIORS

71 ENTERS CALENDAR CODE/LINE AT APPROPRIATE TIME

72 CONFIRMS CALENDAR ENTRY WITH R APPROPRIATELY

73 PRESENTS CAL, SHOWCD OR PHOTOBK AT APPROP TIME

74 DIRECTS R THROUGH THE PHOTOBK APPROPRIATELY

81 FAILS TO ENTER CALENDAR CODE/LINE AT APPROP TIME

82 FAILS TO CONFIRM CAL ENTRY WITH R APPROP

83 FAILS TO PRESENT CAL, SHOWCD OR PHOTOBK AT APPROP TIME

84 FAILS TO DIRECT R THROUGH THE PHOTOBK APPROP

85 ENTERED CALENDAR DATA AT INAPPROPRIATE TIME

86 USES SHOWCARD OR PHOTOBOOK AT INAPPROP TIME

Intro	
A1	
A2	
A3	
A4	
A5	
A6	
A7	
A8	
A9	
A10	

Source: Women's Contraceptive and Reproductive Experiences (CARE) Steering Committee. Women's CARE Study. 1995. US Public Health Service: NICHD and CDC.

Question Number	Correct Skip	No Errors	Minor Errors	Major Errors	Interrupt	Repeat Question	Other Probes	R asks for Clarification
A1		22	2	2				
A1A		25				1	8	
A2		25				5	1	1
A3		22	3				1	
A4		9	11	6		1	1	3
A4A		21	3	1			1	1
A5		24			1			5

Example 39. Compiled Interview Observation Data

Source: Fowler FJ Jr. Improving survey questions: design and evaluation. Sage Publications, Inc., 1995.

Interview behavior coding can be performed quickly by researchers, interviewers, or other study staff with little training *(13)*. Personal pretest interviews can be coded directly by observers, or taped and coded afterward, as they must be for telephone interviews. Videotaping or audio recording is preferred, as it is more objective and provides more credible evidence for findings. Any changes to questions and procedures that are instituted as a result of the first pretest should be carefully examined in the second pretest and tested again if problems persist.

Collecting information from interviewers

This approach involves obtaining information about the tested questions, the elicited answers, and interviewer perceptions about the interview directly from each interviewer. One way to do this is to collect systematic information from each interviewer via questionnaire after the pretest interviews are completed. Question rating forms for interviewers, similar to those shown in previous examples, have been designed and used successfully for this purpose *(13, 79)*. The questions are laid out in table format, and interviewers are asked to assess each

question according to three criteria: its readability, the consistency
with which respondents interpret it, and the consistency with
which respondents are able and willing to answer it. For each crite-
rion, the interviewer responds in one of three ways: no evidence of
problem, possible problem, or definite problem. As with the coding of observed behavior described above, summary tables of all
interviewer findings can be easily created using this scheme.
Another interviewer questionnaire method, which uses a series of
standardized probes to identify questions with potential problems,
is shown in Figure 6.

Figure 6. Standardized probes used for interviewer questionnaire

(1) Did any of the questions seem to make R uncomfortable?

(2) Did you have to repeat any questions?

(3) Did R misinterpret any questions?

(4) Which questions were the most difficult or awkward for you to read? Have you come to
dislike any specific questions? Why?

(5) Did any of the sections seem to drag?

(6) Were there any sections in which you felt that the respondent would have liked the opportunity to say more?

*Source: Converse JM, Presser S. Survey questions: handcrafting the standardized questionnaire. Thousand Oaks, CA
(US): Sage Publications; 1986.*

Interviewers are asked to complete a questionnaire after each
pretest interview and to elaborate on each "Yes" answer by specifying question numbers and providing written explanations. The
quality of information collected via interviewer feedback, regardless
of whether or not the method of collection follows a prescribed
format, depends on the interviewer's ability take copious and accurate margin notes while the interview is taking place, a skill that is
likely to vary considerably between interviewers. Even so, standardized techniques such as those described above are likely to be much
more informative than less structured techniques, such as oral
group debriefing sessions.

Probing respondents

Systematic probing of respondents is carried out with techniques similar to those described under *Phase IIb: Intensive interviews with individual respondents (13)*. Investigators use these probes in questionnaire pretesting when intensive interviews with respondents have not been carried out earlier or when they have lingering doubts about the validity of specific questions in the survey setting. The probes can be built into the pretest to follow specific questions or appended to the end of the questionnaire. Neither approach is ideal since, in the former, the probes risk breaking the flow of the questionnaire and may detract from the ability of the pretest to examine the questionnaire as a whole, and, in the latter, the limitations of respondent memory may decrease the accuracy and completeness of the information reported. In the pretesting of self-administered questionnaires that are mailed to pretest respondents, investigators can include a few of these probing questions as well as more general questions about what the respondent found confusing, for example, although this effort is unlikely to generate useful feedback.

Pretesting of Data Processing Procedures. After the pretest questionnaires have been completed, data should be edited, coded, and prepared for analysis according to standard procedures developed for the study. Data entry software must also be tested. Just as study interviewers should be used to conduct pretest interviews, study personnel should be used to pretest all data processing procedures, including editing, coding, data entry, data tabulation, and all other data-handling tasks. All staff members should be systematically debriefed for any difficulties they may have encountered. Problems that are discovered as a result of feedback and observation, or from review of the tabulated data, should be corrected and reexamined in the next pretest. Constraints on these and all pre-survey evaluation techniques include resources and time. Although the inclusion of these techniques in the study protocol will not ensure accurate and complete data, they have been shown to help minimize measurement error.

Statistical Assessment of Measurement Error. The evaluation techniques described above are designed to identify weaknesses in the questionnaire and its administration that may bias study data if left uncorrected. They do not attempt to quantify the accuracy and precision of the data, however. Such quantitative assessment of validity and reliability can help investigators assess the adequacy of the questionnaire before the instrument is fielded and interpret and generalize study results after the data have been collected *(13, 43)*. Statistical testing is highly recommended, especially for surveys using new instruments or procedures and for surveys using existing protocols in substantially different populations *(43)*. Investigators of large epidemiologic studies may plan experimental pretests with large sample sizes *(43)* that can accomplish these goals, but these can be costly and beyond the budget limitations of smaller studies.

Fortunately, capacity for some statistical assessment of validity or reliability can easily be built into the study questionnaire, or other techniques to measure data quality can be used along with or after primary data collection *(13, 43)*. Statistical tests conducted after the questionnaire is fielded, such as correlational studies and analyses of variance, will enable investigators to estimate the impact of measurement error on study results, make necessary corrections to the results, and offer some information about the generalizability of study results. Although investigators are responsible for considering how well each questionnaire variable corresponds to the true value it purports to measure *(13)*, that is usually a difficult task. To really measure validity, comparisons between the questionnaire variables and error-free measures of the same phenomenon are required. Since error-free measures, or "gold standards," do not exist for the vast majority of questionnaire data, investigators must search for external criteria that are of equal or higher quality than the questionnaire data with which to make comparisons. Although such studies are often called *validity studies (13, 21)*, the term *intermethod reliability*, used by some authors *(43)*, is more accurate. Medical record data, despite their limitations *(13, 64)*, are frequently used to assess the intermethod reliability of questionnaire data. For example, investigators may test the accuracy of breast cancer family history data collected via questionnaire by comparing it with data abstracted from the pathology records of the family members of respondents. Other comparison measures employed by epidemiologists to assess validity via intermethod reliability include physical or biochemical measures of exposure, interviews by experts in the field, exposure diaries, and direct observations (43).

Similarly, intermethod reliability assessment is used to shed light on the predictive validity of questionnaire data by examining how well questionnaire data correlate with related or future events. For example, if certain unhealthy behavior practices are hypothesized to lead to increased use of medical services, persons practicing those behaviors may be expected to have more hospitalizations, doctor visits, or missed work days over time. These outcomes can be measured outside the study and correlated with behavior measured via questionnaire. Aggregate comparisons between questionnaire measures and external measures can also be made *(13)*. For most epidemiologic data collected by questionnaire, however, not only are there no gold standards, but neither are there suitable, external criteria that can be used to assess validity. As a result, investigators commonly measure only the internal consistency or the intramethod reliability of their data to gain information about the validity of their data *(43)*.

Reliability refers to the extent to which similar information is elicited when a measurement is repeated, or a question is asked more than once. When questions are unreliable, respondents are more likely to be misclassified according to key study variables, and this can bias study results. (See Chapter 4: *Epidemiologic Study Design.*) The most common and simplest assay of intramethod reliability in epidemiologic studies is the "test-retest" or "re-interview"study, in which the questionnaire is administered a second time to a subsample of respondents. The two sets of questionnaire responses are compared and assessed. Differences between any pair of responses may be attributable to measurement error or may arise from real changes over time in the phenomenon being measured. Depending on the type of information being collected and the length of time between the two measurements, the true source of the differences may be difficult to identify. A second method to measure the intra-reliability of study data is to repeat selected questions within the questionnaire, using slightly different wording or structure, and then checking for consistency of response *(13, 80)*. One problem with each of these approaches is that, although poorly correlated results will rightly raise concerns about the validity of the study, significant measurement error that is repeated when the questions are repeated or readministered may go unnoticed and unquantified *(43, 81)*.

Despite the difficulties in assessing the reliability and validity of questionnaire data, epidemiologic researchers agree that the process yields critical information about data quality at relatively low cost. Moreover, investigators must continue to search for better methods of validating factual questionnaire data with reliable outside sources. For more subjective epidemiologic data, new methods are needed to evaluate data quality *(13)*. These studies will ultimately lead to better-designed questionnaires and more rigorous, higher quality data. For more in-depth information about the various study designs and analytic techniques used to measure validity and reliability, more detailed sources should be consulted *(43, 81)*.

REFERENCES

1. Jack B, Clarke AM. The purpose and use of questionnaires in research. [Review]. Prof Nurse 1998;14(3):176–9.

2. Kelsey J, Thompson WD, Evans AS. Methods in observational epidemiology. New York, Oxford: Oxford University Press; 1986.

3. Oppenheim AN. Questionnaire design, interviewing, and attitude measurement. New edition. London, New York: Pinter Publishing; 1992.

4. Nunnally JC, Bernstein IH. Psychometric theory. 3rd ed. New York: McGraw-Hill, Inc.; 1994.

5. Posner SF, Pulley L, Artz L, Macaluso M. Use of psychometric techniques in the analysis of epidemiologic data. Ann Epidemiol 2002;13(1):1–7.

6. Fleiss J, Shrout P. The effects of measurement errors on some multivariate procedures. Am J Public Health 1977;67(12):1188–91.

7. Hulley SB, Newman TB, Cummings SR. Getting started: the anatomy and physiology of research. Designing clinical research. Baltimore: Williams & Wilkins; 1988.

8. Greenland S. Basic methods for sensitivity analysis and external adjustment. In: Rothman KJ, Greenland S, editors. Modern epidemiology. Philadelphia: Lippincott-Raven;1998:343–57.

9. Gordis L. Assuring the quality of questionnaire data. Am J Epidemiol 1979;109(1):21–4.

10. Grice HP. Logic and conversation. In: Cole P, Morgan JL, editors. Speech acts. New York: Academic Press; 1975: 41–58.

11. Sudman S, Bradburn NM. Asking questions: a practical guide to questionnaire design. San Francisco: Jossey-Bass; 1982.

12. Clark HH, Schober MF. Asking questions and influencing answers. In: Tanur JM, editor. Questions about questions: inquiries into the cognitive bases of surveys. New York: Russell Sage Foundation, 1992; 15–48.

13. Fowler FJ, Jr. Improving survey questions: design and evaluation. Thousand Oaks, CA: Sage Publications, Inc.; 1995.

14. McDowell I, Newell C. Measuring health: a guide to rating

scales and questionnaires. New York: Oxford University Press; 1996.

15. The United States Code of Federal Regulations (CFR). Title 45 CFR Part 46.401. Available from: http://ohrp.osophs.dhhs.gov/humansubjects/guidance/45cfr46.htm

16. Shamoo AE. Future challenges to human subject protection. The Scientist (online) 2000; 14(13). Accessed December 17, 2001. Available from: http://www.the-scientist.com/yr2000/jun/index_000626.html.

17. Council for International Organizations of Medical Sciences (CIOMS). International Guidelines for Ethical Review of Epidemiologic Studies. Accessed September 1, 2002. Available from: http://www.cioms.ch/frame_guidelines_january_2002.htm.

18. The National Commission for the Protection of Human Subjects of Biomedical and Behavioral Research. The Belmont Report, Office of the Secretary, Ethical Principles and Guidelines for the Protection of Human Subjects of Research. April 18, 1979. DHEW Publication No. (OS) 780013 and No. (OS) 78-0014. U.S. Government Printing Office, Washington, D.C. 20402.

19. The IEA European Epidemiology Group. Good epidemiological practice (GEP): proper conduct in epidemiologic research (Proposal). Accessed November 13, 2001. Available from: http://www.dundee.ac.uk/iea/GoodPract.htm

20. Office for Human Research Protections (OHRP) US Department of Health and Human Services. IRB Guidebook. Accessed June 21, 2001. Available from: http://www.ohrp.osophs.dhhs.gov/references/resource.htm.

21. Bennett AE, Ritchie K. Questionnaires in medicine: a guide to their design and use. London, New York: Oxford University Press for Nuffield Provincial Hospitals Trust; 1975.

22. Schaefer DR, Dillman DA. Development of a standard e-mail methodology—results of an experiment. Public Opin Q 1998;62(3):378–97.

23. Wong K. Database on African Internet Users. Data File, Center for International Development and Conflict Management, University of Maryland.

24. US Department of Commerce. A nation online: how Americans

are expanding their use of the Internet (Executive Summary). Accessed May 14, 2002. Available from: http://www.esa.doc.gov/508/esa/nationonline.htm.

25. Berdie DR, Anderson JF, Niebuhr MA. Questionnaires: design and use. 2nd ed. Metuchen, NJ: Scarecrow Press; 1986.

26. Aday LA. Designing and conducting health surveys: a comprehensive guide. 2nd ed. San Francisco: Jossey-Bass; 1996.

27. Bowling A. Research methods in health: investigating health and health services. Buckingham; Briston, PA: Open University Press; 1997.

28. Nicholls WI, Baker RP, Martin J. The effect of new data collection technologies on survey data. In: Lyberg L, Biemer P, Collins M, de Leeuw E, Dippo C, Schwarz N, et al., editors. Survey measurement and process quality. New York: John Wiley & Sons, Inc.; 1997.

29. Marchbanks PA, McDonald JA, Wilson HG, Burnett NM, et al. The NICHD Women's Contraceptive and Reproductive Experiences Study: methods and operational results. Ann Epidemiol 2002;12:213–21.

30. Slattery ML, Edwards SL, Caan BJ, Kerber RA, Potter JD. Response rates among control subjects in case-control studies. Ann Epidemiol 1995;5(3):245–9.

31. Groves RM, Kahn RL. Surveys by telephone: a national comparison with personal interviews. New York: Academic Press, Inc.; 1979.

32. Rogers TF. Interviews by telephone and in person: quality of responses and field performance. In: Singer E, Presser S, editors. Survey research methods: a reader. Chicago: The University of Chicago Press, 1976; 193–207.

33. Dillman DA. Mail and other self-administered surveys in the 21st century: the beginning of a new era. Gallup Research Journal 1999;2(1):121–40.

34. Trewin D, Lee G. International comparisons of telephone coverage. In: Groves R, Biemer P, Lyberg L, Massey J, Nicholls WI, Waksburg J, editors. Telephone survey methodology. New York: John Wiley & Sons, Inc.; 1988: 9–24.

35. Jobe JB, Pratt WF. Effects of interview mode on sensitive questions in a fertility survey. In: Lyberg L, Biemer P, Collins M, de

Leeuw E, Dippo C, Schwarz N, et al., editors. Survey measurement and process quality. New York: John Wiley & Sons, Inc.; 1997: 311–29.

36. Schoon I. Questionnaire design. In: Nunn J, editor. Laboratory psychology: a beginner's guide. New York: Psychology Press; 1998: 73–96.

37. [Editorial.] The anthrax trail. The Wall Street Journal 2002 Mar 26;Sect. A:22(col. 1).

38. Dillman DA. Mail and telephone surveys; the total design method. New York: Wiley; 1978.

39. Moser CA, Kalton G. Survey methods in social investigation. 2nd ed. New York: Basic Books; 1972.

40. McCarthy GM, MacDonald JK. Nonresponse bias in a national study of dentists' infection control practices and attitudes related to HIV. Community Dent Oral Epidemiol 1997; 25(4):319–23.

41. Green KE. Reluctant respondents: differences between early, late and nonresponders to a mail survey. Paper presented at the Annual Meeting of the American Educational Research Association; 1989 Mar 27–31; San Francisco, California.

42. Strack F, Martin LL. Thinking, judging, and communicating: a process account of context effects in attitude surveys. In: Hippler H-J, Schwarz N, Sudman S, editors. Social information processing and survey methodology. New York: Springer-Verlag, 1987; 123–48.

43. Armstrong BK, White E. Principles of exposure measurement in epidemiology. Oxford, New York: Oxford University Press; 1992.

44. Olsen J. Epidemiology deserves better questionnaires. IEA European Questionnaire Group. International Epidemiological Association. Int J Epidemiol 1998;27(6):935.

45. Converse JM, Presser S. Survey questions: handcrafting the standardized questionnaire. Thousand Oaks, CA (US): Sage Publications, Inc; 1986.

46. McGee J. Collecting information from health care consumers: a resource manual of tested questionnaires and practical advice. Gaithersburg, MD: Aspen Publishers; 1996.

47. Information for Authors. Am J Epidemiol 153 [No. 1]. The School of Hygiene and Public Health, The Johns Hopkins

University; Oxford University Press. Accessed February 27, 2001. Available from: http://www3.oup.co.uk/jnls/list/aje/instauth/auth1.html.

48. Foddy WH. Constructing questions for interviews and question-naires: theory and practice in social research. Cambridge, UK; New York: Cambridge University Press; 1993.

49. Schuman H, Presser S. The open and closed question. Am Sociol Rev 1979; 44(Oct):692–712.

50. Warnecke RB, Johnson TP, Chavez N, Sudman S, O'Rourke DP, Lacey L, et al. Improving question wording in surveys of cultur-ally diverse populations. Ann Epidemiol 1997;7(5):334–42.

51. Women's Contraceptive and Reproductive Experiences (CARE) Steering Committee. Women's CARE Study. US Public Health Service: NICHD and CDC; 1995.

52. Rothman KJ, Greenland S. Measures of disease frequency. In: Rothman KJ, Greenland S, editors. Modern epidemiology. Philadelphia: Lippincott-Raven; 1998: 29–46.

53. Weinberg C, Wilcox AJ. Reproductive epidemiology. In: Rothman KJ, Greenland S, editors. Modern epidemiology. Philadelphia: Lippincott-Raven; 1998: 594.

54. Lehnert WG. The process of question answering. Hillsdale, NJ: Lawrence Erlbaum Associates, Inc.; 1978.

55. Holman CD, Armstrong BK. Hutchinson's melanotic freckle melanoma associated with non-permanent hair dyes. Br J Cancer 1983;48(4):599–601.

56. Cannell CF, Marquis KH, Laurent A, National Center for Health Statistics. A summary of studies of interviewing methodology. Rockville, MD: Health Resources Administration, National Center for Health Statistics; 1977. Vital and Health Statistics, Series 2, No. 69. DHEW Publication No. (HRA) 77-1343.

57. Wingo PA, Ory HW, Layde PM. The evaluation of the data col-lection process for a multicenter, population-based, case-control design. Am J Epidemiol 1988;128:206–17.

58. MACRO International. Demographic Health Survey, Armenia, 1999. Calverton, Maryland: MACRO International; 2001.

59. Serbanescu F, Morris L, Marin M. Reproductive Health Survey: Romania, 1999. Atlanta, GA, Romanian Association of Public

Health and Health Management (ARAPMA); Division of Reproductive Health, Centers for Disease Control and Prevention; US Agency for International Development (USAID); United Nations Population Fund (UNFPA); United Nations Children's Fund (UNICEF). 2001.

60. Anderson B, Silver B, Abramson P. The effects of race of the interviewer on measures of electoral participation by blacks. Public Opin Q 1988;52(1):53–83.

61. Parry HJ, Crossley HM. Validity of responses to survey questions. Public Opin Q 1950;14(61):80.

62. Fox JA, Tracy PE. Randomized response: a method for sensitive surveys. Beverly Hills: Sage Publications; 1986.

63. Armstrong BK, White E, Saracci R. The design of questionnaires. Principles of exposure measurement in epidemiology. London, New York: Oxford University Press; 1992.

64. Cannell CF, Miller P, Oksenberg L. Research on interviewing techniques. In: Leinhardt S, editor. Sociological methodology. San Francisco: Jossey-Bass; 1981: 389–437.

65. Cannell CF. Experiments in the improvement of response accuracy. In: Beed TW, Stimson RJ, editors. Survey interviewing—theory and techniques. Sydney: George Allen and Unwin; 1985: 24–62.

66. Sudman S, Bradburn NM, Schwarz N. Thinking about answers: the application of cognitive processes to survey methodology. San Francisco: Jossey-Bass, Inc.; 1996.

67. Jobe JB, Mingay DJ. Cognitive research improves questionnaires. Am J Public Health 1989;79(8):1053–55.

68. Wanke M, Schwarz N. Reducing question order effects: the operation of buffer items. In: Lyberg L, Biemer P, Collins M, de Leeuw E, Dippo C, Schwarz N, et al., editors. Survey measurement and process quality. John Wiley & Sons, Inc.; 1997:115.

69. Schwarz N. Judgement in a social context: biases, shortcomings, and the logic of conversation. Advances in Experimental Social Psychology 1994;26:123–62.

70. Schuman H, Presser S, Ludwig J. Context effects on survey responses to questions about abortion. Public Opin Q 1981;45(2):216–23.

71. Jenkins CR, Dillman DA. Towards a theory of self-administered questionnaire design. In: Lyberg L, Biemer P, Collins M, de Leeuw E, Dippo C, Schwarz N et al., editors. Survey measurement and process quality. New York: John Wiley & Sons, Inc.; 1997: 165–96.

72. Lee JA, More SJ, Cotiw-an BS. Problems translating a questionnaire in a cross-cultural setting. Prev Vet Med 1999; 41 (2-3):187–94.

73. Gille H, van de Kaa DJ. Contributions of the World Fertility Survey to survey methodology and analysis. NIDI Reprint Series no. 24. Voorburg, Netherlands: Netherlands Interuniversity Demographic Institute [NIDI];1983:21.

74. Johnson T, O'Rourke D, Chavez N, Sudman S, Warneke R, Lacey L, et al. Social cognition and responses to survey questions among culturally diverse populations. In: Lyberg L, Biemer P, Collins J, de Leeuw E, Dippo C, Schwarz N, et al., editors. Survey measurement and process quality. New York: John Wiley & Sons, Inc.; 1997: 87–113.

75. Del Greco L, Walop W. Questionnaire development: 3. Translation. CMAJ 1987;136(10):1025–6.

76. Forsyth BH, Lessler JT. Cognitive laboratory methods: a taxonomy. In: Biemer P, Groves RM, Lyberg L, Mathiowetz NA, Sudman S, editors. Measurement errors in surveys. New York: John Wiley & Sons; 1991.

77. Lessler J, Tourangeau R, Salter W, National Center for Health Statistics. Questionnaire design in the cognitive research laboratory. Rockville, MD: National Center for Health Statistics; 1989.

78. Cannell CF, Lawson SA, Hausser DL. A technique for evaluating interviewer performance. Ann Arbor MI: Survey Research Center, Institute for Social Research, The University of Michigan; 1975.

79. Oksenberg L, Cannell CF, Kalton G. New strategies for testing survey questions. J Off Stat 1991;7:349–65.

80. Stolley PD, Schlesselman JJ. Planning and conducting a study. In: Schlesselman JJ, editor. Case-control studies: design, conduct analysis. New York: Oxford University Press; 1982: 69–104.

81. Andrews FM. Construct validity and error components of survey measure: a structural modeling approach. In: Singer E, Presser S, editors. Survey research methods: a reader. Chicago: University of Chicago Press; 1989: 391–425.

QUESTIONNAIRE DEVELOPMENT EXERCISES

Exercise 1: Critique an existing questionnaire (individual exercise)

The questionnaire should be one designed to collect information from individuals, as opposed to medical records, for example. It may be designed to be self-administered or administered by an interviewer, and for research or surveillance purposes. A fully developed draft of a new questionnaire would also be acceptable.

1. How will the questionnaire be administered?

2. What measures have been taken to protect the identity and privacy of respondents who complete the questionnaire?

3. Describe the formatting and layout of the questionnaire. Has it been designed to maximize data quality? How could it be improved? Comment on the overall appearance of the questionnaire.

4. Describe the specific purpose of the questionnaire, including the specific research question(s) that will be answered from the collected data.

5. Choose one of these research questions. List all of the variables that will be required to answer this question, including any confounding variables and possible effect modifiers that will have to be examined. Describe which questions will be used to create each of those variables, how they will be coded, and all units of measurement.

6. How will missing values be handled?

7. Is there a need to separate unknown responses from refusals? If so, how will responses be coded to facilitate this?

8. How will unanticipated responses be handled?

9. Carefully consider the wording of each of these questions. How well has the intent of each question been communicated? Does each question specify the way in which it should be answered? Are some respondents likely to be unable or unwilling to answer any of these questions? What measures, if any, have been taken to ensure that these questions are administered in the same way to all respondents?

10. Consider the order of the questions in the questionnaire. How likely is it that previous questions could bias responses to questions that follow? Can you suggest a better order for the questions?

11. What safeguards, if any, have been built into the questionnaire to help ensure validity of the data?

Exercise 2: Develop a draft of a questionnaire (team exercise)

The instructor/class decides on a research question and target population. The class divides into teams, which are given the following tasks, one at a time. After each task is completed or the allotted time has been spent, teams report on their results, and discussion follows.

1. What is the best type of questionnaire for this study and how, exactly, should it be administered?

    a) Assume study budget is robust. Given what you know about the purpose of the study and the target population, describe the ideal methods of contacting subjects and collecting information; include all technology that will be used.

    b) Assume study budget is severely limited. Under these circumstances, and considering what you know about the purpose of the study and the target population, describe an alternative methodology to contact subjects and collect information. Describe the strengths and limitations of these methods in comparison to those described in a).

2. Assume you have reviewed the literature and have decided against borrowing questions from an existing questionnaire to measure the primary exposure variable.

    a) What are some reasons investigators may choose to design their own questions?

    b) Draft the questions you propose to use to measure this exposure, including any visual memory aids you will use, and describe all Phase I and Phase II activities you will use to evaluate them.

    c) Have you opted to use open questions, closed questions, or a combination of open and closed questions, and why?

    d) What are some possible weaknesses of the questions you have drafted, and how, specifically, will you assess these concerns?

e) Draft a "double interview" between interviewer and respondent that will address these concerns.

3. Format the questions and describe how this formatting will facilitate consistent administration of the questions, consistent coding, and consistent data entry.

4. Describe your plans to pretest your questionnaire, including respondent contact, data collection, and data processing procedures. Sample size, characteristics of the pretest subjects, procedures to further evaluate exposure questions described in 2b), procedures to collect data from interviewers (if used), and other planned activities should be described.

5. Describe your plans to statistically assess the validity of your data.

www.ingramcontent.com/pod-product-compliance
Lightning Source LLC
Chambersburg PA
CBHW081845170526
45167CB00007B/2909